Walter Lübeck

Aura Healing Handbook

Learn to Read and Interpret the Aura
Perceive Energy Fields in Color and
Utilize Them for Holistic Healing

Astrology and New Age Series No. 2

Walter Lübeck

Aura Healing Handbook

Learn to Read and Interpret the Aura
Perceive Energy Fields in Color and
Utilize Them for Holistic Healing

Translated by Christine M. Grimm

Sri Satguru Publications
A Division of
Indian Books Centre
Delhi, India

Published by
Sri Satguru Publications,
Indological and Oriental Publishers
A Division of
Indian Books Centre
40/5, Shakti Nagar,
Delhi-110007
India

Email: ibcindia@vsnl.com
Website: http://www.indianbookscentre.com

First Indian Edition; Delhi, 2000

ISBN 81-7030-686-8

Published by Sunil Gupta for Sri Satguru Publications, a division of Indian Books Centre, 40/5, Shakti Nagar, Delhi-110007, India and printed at Chawla Offset Printers, Delhi 110 052

DEDICATION

For Manuela

Table of Contents

Acknowledgements

I needed a great many impulses in order to write this book. I would like to express especially heartfelt thanks to some of the people who helped me on my path:

My parents for their openness, love, and the curiosity and zest for life that they gave me on my way. My fairy and my Higher Self for protection and understanding of my many large and small weaknesses and their constant encouragement to keep going. Brigitte Müller, my Reiki Master who triggered some initial changes within me. Renate Lorke and Wolfgang Grabowski, who helped me deal with my spiritual experiences in a meaningful way. Elke Erdmann for her example of how to approach clairvoyance in a practical way. And last but not least, my good friend Manuela for her understanding, the mirror, her love, and... and....

Foreword

The aura is an energy field around the body of a life form. This means that human beings, animals, plants, minerals, etc. all have an aura. Since most people unfortunately only use a portion of their senses (eyes, ears, nose, hands, mouth, and subtle senses), they generally don't see this field. However, each individual has been given this ability. A bit of training and practice are necessary.

I would like to give you an example from another sensory area: I had a color and individual type consultation done for myself. A white cloth was put around my shoulders and I sat in front of a mirror without any makeup. One after the other, solid-colored scarves were placed around my shoulders. Then I was asked to pay close attention to my face, particularly my eyes, my mouth, my skin coloring, etc. At first I couldn't discover any change in my face when the color changed. However, after some time my eyes became used to this kind of seeing and I now could determine the changes. With some colors, my face was pale or my skin looked leathery. In turn, other colors emphasized my eyes or my mouth. Now I had learned to see in an expanded way. As I said, at first my eyes had to get used to "seeing" in this different way. Some people would perhaps even call this seeing with other eyes, although they still are my own eyes.

The situation is similar in terms of professions. If someone deals with figures every day, then he will not only have a good memory for figures but can also much more quickly recognize errors than a person who doesn't deal with them as frequently. He will already see at first glance when a number simply doesn't fit, which means that his eyes are trained to see things or not see them. Why shouldn't we take full advantage of the capacity of our eyes when this is possible for us? There's nothing different about seeing the aura. We can all learn to perceive even more than we did before. This book provides some ideas and suggestions as to how this type of training can be accomplished. I personally find it very exciting to discover new things. At first, when I started to see the energy bodies and the chakras, I couldn't believe it. I thought I was just imagining everything. Yet, when the confirmations came I was amazed and simply had to believe it. At the start I could only see darkly, then I could also see somewhat lighter tones—everything in gray tones like dark gray, medium gray, etc. Perhaps I will soon also be able to see in color.

But this doesn't mean that I walk along the street and always see the chakras of all the people I pass. Instead, I can look when I want to and don't have to see them otherwise. I only use this new ability when someone asks me to do so. It would be terrible if I couldn't switch it on and off.

I wish you much enjoyment in trying out and experimenting with the contents of this book. It's great when there's something new to discover time and again. It's great when this isn't boring. It's great when you have the courage to see.

Manuela Lübeck

Introduction

Reading auras and developing my subtle senses have a very significant personal meaning for me. I have so many things that I owe to these abilities that it's hard for me to imagine my way of life without them. For example, I met my wife and long-standing companion in life through them. One evening many years ago, I asked to be led to the appropriate partner and then simply followed the guidance of my sixth sense...

Many important professional decisions can be made by using these abilities so that all participants benefit from them. Among other things, I attribute my relatively easy access to subtle perceptions to the fact that I surrendered the guidance for my personality's development to the powers of love and light during my first independent contacts with the spiritual world and made an intensive effort to learn to perceive and interpret their messages in the following time period.

The reason for my easy access to this type of perception was probably based on an experience many years ago that influenced my entire path in life. As a small child, I came into contact with beings from the subtle plane while I played in the sandbox. When you have experienced something like this, you no longer need to think about whether or not there's something to be learned in the spiritual realm and how to approach this in the future. Afterwards, some years passed before I once again had direct contact with esoteric things. However, my parents had and still have a very open attitude toward this area of life. This meant that I came into contact with it time and again in a completely incidental and quite natural and practical way. Their stories made it easier for me to comprehend the use of the "sixth sense" and confirmed its existence for me. Conversations on these topics in our home weren't concerned with whether something like this existed or not, but rather what my parents and their ancestors had experienced with it. For example, my father survived both world wars only because of premonitions. In quite an incidental way, I therefore heard fascinating stories from their lives about hypnosis, telepathy, clairvoyance, astrology, and folk magic. With the curiosity of a child, I took in everything. In time I began to strive for further experiences of my own in this area.

During puberty, I became interested in using the pendulum and radiesthesia. Later, I also got involved with many other areas of esoteric knowledge. Tao Yoga and Tai Chi Chuan, the I Ching, and Tarot became my good friends and companions that I wouldn't want to do without today.

Yet, I wasn't permitted a direct view of the subtle planes until I received the Second Reiki Degree* at the age of twenty-seven.

A few months after the Second Degree seminar, I noticed a new type of perceptive ability within myself, which I had previously just heard of and read about: In my inner eye I could see where other people's vital energy was congested and where it flowed. The blocks looked black or dark, and the areas in which the vital energy flowed well were light or clear. At first I couldn't really trust this new sense, yet the more frequently my insights into the subtle planes were confirmed, the more I valued my perceptions. I tried out the inner vision time and again and then noticed that I could also observe animals and plants, and even minerals, in this way.

Since I basically have a skeptical nature, I checked my observations in a great variety of ways again and again and tried to bring them into harmony with my knowledge about energetic and anatomic correlations. I spent many hours browsing through bookstores in search of literature that could help me interpret what I saw. Then I also noticed time and again that I could was quite capable of perceiving what wasn't "in balance," although it was hard for me to recognize the issue at hand and what effects a certain block could have on the life and health of the respective person.

Along the same lines, I couldn't exactly determine on which level I was seeing something at the moment. Sometimes these were congested places that later turned out to be in the physical area (for example, scars), sometimes in the emotional area (for example, the anger to which someone was clinging), or in the area of the chakras and meridians. The energetic levels were often mixed with each other so that I saw blocked sorrow and bodily zones with poor circulation together, for example. My experiences with Tao Yoga and

---

* Reiki is an ancient energetic art of healing, which was rediscovered in our age by the Japanese Dr. Mikao Usui. The ability to work with Reiki can be conveyed from an empowered Reiki Master to any other person through initiations. Also see the bibliography.

acupuncture made it possible for me to discover some things, but others simply couldn't be explained in this way.

The numerous books on the aura, the chakras, and the interpretation of clairvoyant observations confused me more than they helped me. There was no book in which I could read something about a "black-and-white" clairvoyance as I had seen it. It almost appeared as if no author who had written about reading auras was familiar with this expression of clairvoyance, which made me feel insecure about it.

At times I thought there might possibly be something wrong with me and that I was having hallucinations. Yet, my energy-field readings, as I now called my way of seeing the aura, were confirmed time and again by other people. So it couldn't just be nonsense either.

Moreover, there were many contradictions in the books. One said that a human being's aura has three layers, others said it had seven, and even others listed nine. There was even a greater variety of opinions about the number, position, and function of the chakras. The same applied to the classification and interpretation of the colors. For example, the Theosophists generally agreed with each other, but this didn't necessarily correspond with the Chinese, Tibetan, or Native American sources. All of the authors claimed to possess immense experience and great knowledge about subtle states and supported their claims with impressive reports meant to prove the practical applicability of their methods.

Time and again I also read and heard from other people interested in esotericism that clairvoyants are illuminated human beings: blessed with great wisdom and a direct line to God. On the other hand, through my involvement in dowsing, I have experienced that completely "normal" mortals achieve excellent results in using their subtle senses. So the subtle perceptiveness couldn't just be reserved for saints, which made me very happy since I wasn't one and there was still a chance that my strange perceptions had a basis in reality.

Later, when I was the publisher of an esoterically oriented regional magazine, I occasionally had contacts with people who said that they were clairvoyant. I heard some fantastic things from them. When looking at another individual's aura, they saw this person's future, recognizing personal difficulties and karmic burdens. Some of them even discovered outside entities in the auras and described

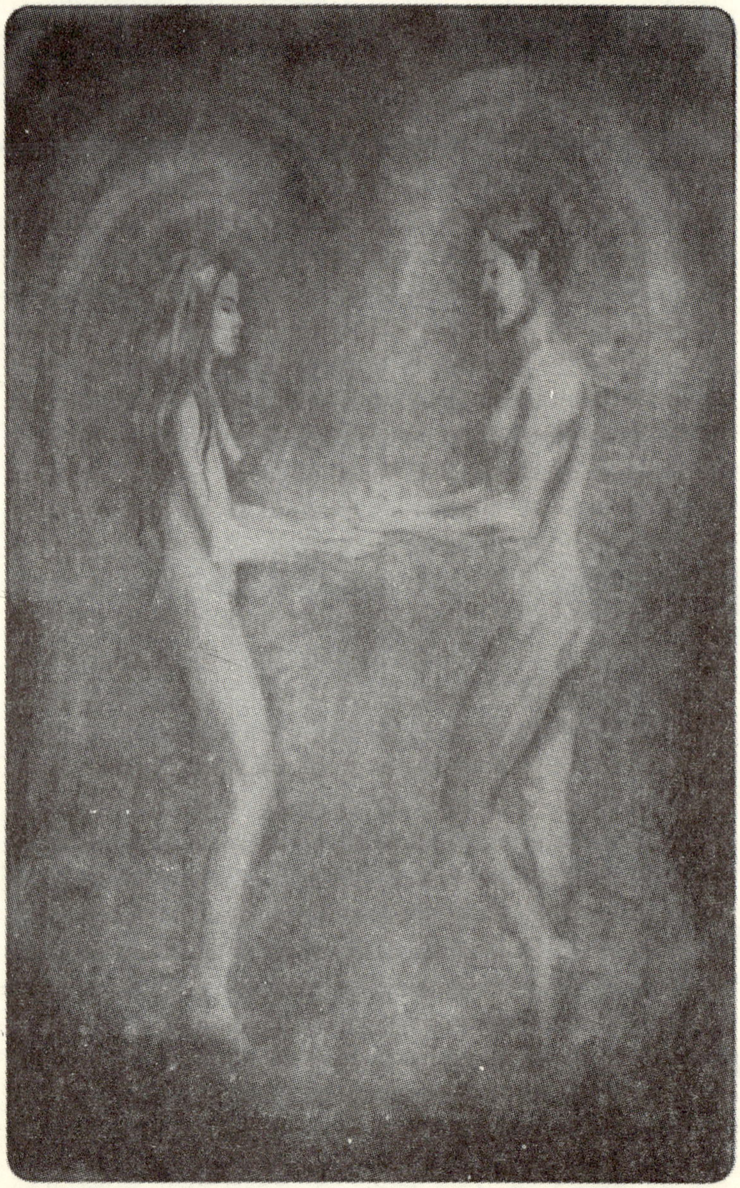

Feeling with the six senses

their past and the reasons why these lost souls were bound to the respective people. This naturally fascinated me very much, and I began to explore whether I could also somehow perceive these things.

But what still very much irritated me was the fact that almost every person gave a different description of the subtle world here as well, even though many of these clairvoyants were completely successful and greatly beneficial to the people who sought them for advice and help.

After I had come into contact with so many types of subtle sensory perception, I began to systematically do research for myself in order to find my own way. For support I looked to a teacher who had always proven to be objective and trustworthy for me: some years before I had rather coincidentally discovered that the ancient Chinese Book of Changes, the I Ching, actually contained a very detailed description of the chakra system. I now made use of this knowledge and explored the tasks and functions of the human body's main energy centers together with the I Ching. In doing so, I discovered that it's not only possible to ask questions of the I Ching with coins and yarrow stalks, but that a simple exercise without any external aids allowed me to determine the state of my chakras. Because of my black-and-white clairvoyant abilities, I could also use this method to read other people's chakras. Now I could quickly and precisely determine a person's energetic state in relation to a specific question and interpret it on the basis of the I Ching (also see Chapter 6: Reading and Interpreting Energy Fields with the I Ching).

In the course of time, I was able to use this method for checking certain prevailing opinions about the function, position, and tasks of the individual chakras, among other things. For example, this confirmed my observation that there aren't any fixed rotational directions in the male and female chakras, but that these change constantly within the overall context of the organism in relation to the demands placed on them. The greater my understanding of the energetic relationships within the body, the deeper and more differentiated my clairvoyance also became. I learned to switch between the individual levels and separate the important things from the unimportant. The more I worked with the I Ching on the interpretation of my observations, the better I could put my abilities to use.

After my successes had encouraged me, I began to also become interested in color clairvoyance and develop my abilities in this direction. This helped me to have further experiences and perceptions that were very interesting and important for my personal development.

Within the scope of my Reiki courses (I've been a Reiki Master for some years now), time and again I encountered people who I found to have abilities similar to my own. When we talked about our experiences in this area, I discovered that they just were just as interested in having support in dealing with their ability as I was. This is where the idea for this book originated. I made the effort of creating a type of course that starts with the "ABCs." From the restoration of the body's ability to resonate, the centering within the HARA, to black-and-white clairvoyance, reading the chakras with the I Ching, and up to the color perception of all energy levels, each element is built upon the one before it. It's very important here to start "at the bottom" and not just page through the last chapter, then look at the cat to see its chakras in color, and, if that doesn't work, throw the book into the recycling box in disappointment. The way you learn the basics will particularly influence whether you really derive a benefit for yourself and others from the wonderful abilities of directly perceiving the energetic level. For this reason, it would be in your interest to read the beginning section of this book, even if you're already an "old hand," and carefully do the exercises. By the way, there will also be some interesting and exciting surprises for you in the first section. If you don't yet know much about esotericism, you can get a solid basis for yourself in the section on the basics. I have limited myself to explaining just the most important terms of esoteric jargon within this context so that reading is more fun for you. On the back side of the book cover, there are some sample colors to make it easier for you to interpret your color perceptions. This will help you understand what colors and color tones are meant when we work with reading the aura in color.

The system and the exercises in this book have been put to the practical test, tried out, and applied in many thousands of cases by myself and hundreds of students during the past years. So they work. If you should at some point have difficulties with the individual learning steps and exercises, be patient with yourself. The truism that Rome wasn't built in a day has much truth to it.

And the patience, humility, and love that you will quite automatically develop in once again permitting subtle perceptions (because otherwise nothing in this area will truly function) will perhaps in retrospect appear to you to be even more significant abilities than the direct access to the subtle world once you have rediscovered it. In any case, that's how I experience it.

And now I wish you much enjoyment in our mutual journey of discovery into the subtle world.

Chapter 1

Why Should I Learn to Read Auras?

Yes, what's this actually all about? Isn't there enough to discover with our normal five senses? We don't even take full advantage of our possibilities of perception as it is!

Absolutely right. However, in my opinion, every sense is worth consideration. The more possibilities I have of perceiving the world, the more easily I can open up to it and decide on the basis of my personal responsibility what's good for me and what isn't; I can learn to more easily accept myself and my feelings and understand the significance of my relationships with others. As long as I'm dependent on second-hand information, I can never learn to find and accept my own path in life. The opinions of others will shape my life since I don't have a solid foundation for my own standpoint. And since there are as many opinions as there are people, I will increasingly lose myself with time as I search for a person who can finally tell me what's right and wrong for me. Yet, each of us has everything available that we need in order to see our own path is and to walk it. This is why it's important for me to discover my abilities and recognize their value.

Once I have had experiences with my diverse possibilities of perception, I then place an emphasis at some point. However, I must first become familiar with all the possibilities.

This book will give you ample ideas for experiencing clairvoyance. Try them out thoroughly and then decide whether you want to further develop these abilities.

There are many new things to discover. New, previously unknown levels of life and experience are waiting for you. Have you ever seen how the energy of a medication shows up in a person's aura when you hold it close to him or her? Or how a colored cloud of energy streams from your partner's heart chakra when he or she gives you a loving look? You can learn to judge the quality of your food and drink in terms of its vital energy in a simple way by observing its emanations. In order to find earth rays, you usually don't need a dowsing rod or a pendulum once you have had some experience with clairvoyance. You can even see the polarity of an earth ray when you practice this ability. It's often said that people in our age have forgotten how to look for stress-creating rays in their living space with dowsing rods and pendulums. I believe that these aids only became necessary when our ancestors no longer permitted themselves to view things directly. Animals don't have any dowsing rods either and can still safely find the places that are energetically correct for them.

Since I have learned to once again open up to my clairvoyance, I have developed a completely different way of dealing with the world. In the past, I used to frequently search for the right information, the competent expert, or the most appropriate system of esotericism. Today, through the possibility of direct perception in the energetic field, I've learned to discover the information that is right for me on my own and adapt for myself the esoteric system that basically fits my personality and explore it. This saves me much time and energy and I always get what's right for me in the holistic sense. I only have to keep my eyes open and assume responsibility for my development.

I would like to tell you a little story related to the esoteric systems that people believe to be generally valid. I sometimes find that these are very obstructive to the process of becoming conscious because of their many laws and ways of labelling things:

In a distant land, far removed from our world, a long time ago there lived a nation of people who were basically just like we are today. They were capable of everything that we can also do today, with one exception—they were incapable of seeing. At some point in the course of time, they had lost this ability. Yet, some of them still knew about sight, and they had the deep desire to once again learn to see the colors of the world. Now and then, rumors came to this nation from far off lands about people who could see. Some of them believed these stories, but others laughed at the nonsense since they didn't know anyone who could see. So these tales couldn't be true, they thought. Those who believed these stories collected all the rumors and news about sight that came to their ears, and some of them even distinguished themselves as teachers of seeing over time. These people had collected so much information about sight and colors that they could give exact explanations to others who didn't know as much as they did about how ripe bananas are always yellow. They had namely heard a story about someone who could see in which ripe, yellow bananas had been mentioned. Since this information came from someone gifted with sight, as the respectable teachers of sight confirmed, it had to be right. And from this time forth, the dogma that ripe bananas are yellow was considered valid. However, at another school of sight, there was a deviating opinion. The teacher who headed this school had namely gathered from another story that ripe bananas are brown. Since he trusted his source more than that of the other school, he established the doctrine that ripe bananas have a brown color. Yet, since he was a tolerant person, he included the teachings of the other school in his system and maintained that only highly developed people with vision could perceive a ripe banana as brown. Those who were not as advanced saw mature bananas in the color yellow. But they still had the possibility of giving up their imperfection at some point and joining his school.

Both of these schools existed for many years. However, several generations of students had become teachers in the meantime and, after their deaths, had made room for other students who had become teachers. These teachers now claimed that they could see. Perhaps this was even true, but how could their abilities be examined? They knew so much about the world of colors that they could classify anything by heart according to the color established by a previous teacher. And since they earned their living on the basis of their work at a certain school of sight, and were also shown affection and respect by students because of their affiliation with the respective famous school, those who had genuinely learned to see had understandable reasons for imparting their teacher's opinions in an unchanged form and maintaining the comfortable system rather than questioning it. Many of them were more concerned with the ethical and moral progress made by their students than the ability to see in itself. They considered the path of learning to see as a possibility for character development and less as a method for truly learning to see.

Since no one could check up them, they taught according to their own system and frequently debated with other teachers about their opinions, indulging in subtle discussions on the world of colors. In the meantime, there were occasionally a few individuals who could see something. They hadn't done anything to achieve this: they had simply been born with the ability. Since they looked for other like-minded people, they soon came into contact with the schools of sight and were welcomed there as new students. But not for long. Whenever they said something about what they saw, the others became frightened because their sight didn't correlate exactly with what the teachings described. And soon they were driven out of the schools as heretics so that the purity of the true teachings would remain intact. Some of the people capable of seeing changed schools since they believed at the start that they had just entered the wrong school. The members of the other schools naturally supported them in this opinion. However, things went just as badly for them there as before at the first school. Tired and confused by all the conflicts, many of them distanced themselves from the schools in general and declared that sight corrupted human beings. Others lets themselves be talked into renouncing their own abilities. From that time on they interpreted what they saw as dictated by the respective school. These people were simply weary of being lonely, and it was easier for them to conform their own perceptions to the teachings than to live without friends.

A very few of those who could actually see no longer spoke to the others about their perceptions. They had been injured too frequently to want to continue fighting about it. Sometimes these people who could see and had gone underground secretly accepted students and tried to convey to them what they knew; yet, their students usually ridiculed them after some time because what they were expected to learn was too much in contradiction to what the great and famous schools taught.

So much for the fairy tale. Does it sound familiar? Well, things aren't quite that dramatic in the spiritual scene today!?! However, in earlier times, such as during the long years when people were burned as witches and sorcerers, having the "wrong" view of the world sometimes had a deadly effect. And we still are trying to deal with this heritage in many respects today.

If you learn to "see" on your own, you can have many rather safe experiences with the subtle world and develop an understanding of the Creation that isn't based on theories.

I find the emotional level to be a very interesting area for applying the ability of seeing auras. It's exciting to watch how emotional energies flow out of and into the various areas of the body, and then observe with the "normal" senses how these forces express themselves in terms of behavior. I often work on this level during the personal counseling sessions that I give. In this way, it's easy to determine whether what my client tells me harmonizes with his or her feelings or whether it comes from the intellectual level. Since a dissonance between these two levels is one of the main sources for problems in life, this approach can provide quick and effective support here. When two people who have difficulties with each other come for counseling together, an aura reading on the emotional level can also be quite helpful. Usually both of them are unaware of where the problem that they have with each other actually is. However, a little "checkup" of the various levels of the relationship allows us to close in on the problem field. In this area, reading auras can be particularly useful for psychotherapists of all schools in order to more easily work through to the heart of the matter when well-being is disrupted. But a physician or healing practitioner can also profit greatly from this ability.

In addition to the usual examination, a checkup by way of looking at the aura can show whether a health disorder actually has a physical cause and where its roots are located, or whether the reasons tend to be psychosomatic. For healers in all fields who work on the energetic level, seeing the aura reveals a great deal more so that they have perceived the bodily zones that energy work is good at reaching and can also immediately examine the effect of the energetic treatment.

In case you aren't a "professional," but just want to learn to read auras for your own personal use, you can probably make the best use of it with respect to your personal development. Every time you use this ability, you will get a deep insight into the subtle world of energies. Here you can see, directly and without illusions, what you are like and how you relate to other people, animals, plants, minerals, medications, and so forth.

The more you perceive of yourself, the more opportunities you will have of recognizing your blind spots, the unloved and unresolved portions of your personality, and find ways to integrate them. The more you are in harmony with yourself, the healthier and more fulfilled you will spend your lifetime here on earth. Then you will be on the path of light and live love.

Seeing auras can also help you in everyday life to better deal with relationships. You will be more likely to see the true issues in a relationship with a colleague, your partner in life, or a friend. This will help you tune in better to the issues involved. You can often already determine health problems in yourself and others during their energetic development, at a time in which they cannot be recognized with the usual methods of diagnosis or only with great effort. So it's possible to take preventive measures in a way that's usually quite simple, not even allowing a serious illness in the physical or psychological area even occur. Consciousness makes life and learning easier.

If you are involved with exercises that promote your development, like Yoga, Qi Gong, or the Five Tibetans, by using certain methods of seeing the aura you can determine in an easy way whether the exercises have the described effect on you. You no longer have to depend on teachings that may or may not apply to you. This puts you in the position of assuming responsibility for yourself and acting in an independent way.

You can even create your own exercises and breathing methods with the help of direct subtle perception. These exercises will then be custom-made for your current condition and your personality.

All of this is just a small excerpt of the possibilities that the various methods of reading the aura offer to you. The practice starts right away in the next chapter. But first you should make a contract with yourself.

About Responsibility

Every human being fundamentally has the ability to see auras. How much access to this ability you achieve basically depends on two things:

1. Do you want to learn it?
2. Can you plausibly guarantee your subconscious mind/Inner Child that you will not harm yourself or anyone else as a result of using this ability, but that you will help yourself and others in the development toward light and love when you use it?

The first condition is quite simple to fulfill and I don't think I need to comment on it. The situation is different for the second. Some explanations are necessary in order to show you the importance of this condition. The Inner Child is the part of an individual's personality that has direct access to extrasensory perception and abilities of all types. It has quite a fixed concept of morality in relation to the use of these abilities. These moral concepts are somewhat different for every human being. However, they do have a common root since the issue at hand is always not harming one's own self and not harming other people. If your Inner Child becomes convinced that you want to treat your spiritual abilities in a way that is willing to oblige and be responsible, it won't have anything against opening the door to the astral world a bit at the start. If you continue to prove yourself trustworthy, you will receive more insights.

But if you're at the beginning at the moment, this is "just" a matter of getting a relatively clear look at the world of energies and subtle powers.

The Inner Child will block the development of these abilities as long as you (the Middle Self/your conscious portion) haven't made it completely clear that you fundamentally don't want to cause any damage.

So that things can get off to a start, please carry out the following little ritual (rituals are a language that your Inner Child understands well!) and approach it seriously, even if your intellect might find it to be silly at the moment.

Later we will look at the various parts of the personality—the Inner Child/Middle Self/Higher Self—and go into their significance in the overall context of your personality.

The ritual: Set aside a good hour of your time to do this. Fill the bathtub and perfume the water with a few drops of sandalwood oil (natural origin!). Take a bath, washing yourself thoroughly and consciously. Perceive the water and the fragrance of the oil. Surrender to the relaxation and enjoy the pleasant warmth around you. When you wash yourself, become aware that you are leaving the things of everyday life behind and removing disruptive vibrations from your aura. Rinse yourself off with lukewarm water at the end. Then wrap yourself in a comfortable bathrobe, take a blanket, and go to a room in which you can remain undisturbed for a while. Stand with bare feet, legs about one-and-a-half shoulder-widths apart. Lift your arms to the heavens, bend your knees somewhat, and raise your face a bit. Perceive the ground beneath your feet, which always securely supports you and permits the feeling that you are in unity with other parts of the Creation. Remain with this feeling for a few breaths. Then direct your attention to the sky above the top of your head, from which life energies constantly flow into you and attempt to support your development. Also perceive the contact with these energies for a few breath cycles. Now direct your attention to the flow of your breath. Each time you inhale, visualize the light stream of heavenly energy that flows into you through the top of your head and fills your body from head to foot.

Every time you exhale, let a stream of dark Earth energy flow into you through your feet and fill you completely. Repeat this breathing exercise at least thirty times. It will balance your body energies and help you come into contact with your Inner Child. Now stand up straight and light three candles—a light-colored one for your Higher Self, a dark one for your Inner Child, and a violet one for the conscious, rational part of your personality, your Middle Self. Now you just need to light some sandalwood incense (the aroma of which will relax you and foster the communication with your Inner Child), then the final portion of the ritual can begin: making and signing a contract with yourself.

Take a blank piece of paper, perhaps handmade paper, in order to also optically highlight the significance of this document. Please write with violet ink or a pen with a violet color. When everything is ready, put your hands on your lap for a moment, close your eyes, feel how you are breathing, and say quietly: "I am at my center, I am with myself and will now enter into a new, wonderful phase of my life through my clear and distinct decision!"

Now take the paper and pen and write:

Contract

I, (your complete name), born on ... at (time, if known), in (place), irrevocably and of my own free will declare herewith that I will use all the spiritual powers to which I gain access only for the best of all those involved. I will respect the freedom of all beings when I put these abilities to use and only do so with their consent in relation to them. I call upon you, you high powers of light and love, to be witnesses and guardians of this contract and ask you to support me in my efforts, to help me when I need help, and to advise me when I need advice in order to fulfill my intention in life.

I hereby irrevocably dedicate my spiritual development to the universal powers of light and love and gratefully and respectfully accept their protection and care.

(Place, date)

(Your signature)

It doesn't matter if you make mistakes in writing it. That doesn't influence your promise.

Pick up the paper with your written promise, breathe on it three times, and let your breath stream out of your heart while you do this. This will help you to accept this promise on all three levels of your personality.

Afterwards, roll up the document and bind it with a white, a black, and a violet ribbon (for example, gift ribbon or silk ribbon). You shouldn't fold or bend it. Keep the document in a safe place. By "safe" I mean that it shouldn't get dirty or bent. Go ahead and show it to other people if you have a good feeling about doing so. After this little ritual, stay with yourself for another moment and feel what's going on inside yourself. If you like, celebrate your vow alone or with friends afterwards. You have reason enough to do so since you have given yourself and the rest of the world a wonderful gift. In no case should you go back to hectic activities right after this ritual. If you don't feel like celebrating, then take a walk in the woods. In any case, give yourself the opportunity to calmly work through all of this, to intregrate it and perceive yourself in your new state, blessed by the powers of light and love.

Chapter 2

Returning into Full Resonance

In my system, the first step to regaining the ability of subtle perception is learning to allow bodily resonance. This means perceiving the vibration of your own body and how it changes through the vibrating energy fields of the surrounding world.

Everything Has Vibrations

All the matter, of which our world is made, vibrates—even crystals, although they appear hard and inflexible to us. These qualities are used in quartz clocks, for example, to measure time. Human beings, animals, plants, minerals, water—all these things constantly move in various rhythms, composed of their respective individual rhythm and their resonance to the vibrations of their environment. The esoteric tradition has been aware of these laws for thousands of years. Modern physics has been able to confirm this ancient knowledge in recent decades through systematic research. For example, there is now knowledge about the structure of matter proving that all atoms and subatomic particles of a substances are involved in constant, very fast movement. In reality, what we believe to recognize as solid matter is actually a collection of many tiny particles moving so quickly that we get the impression of a solid body. You can get an idea of this effect by watching an airplane propeller as it starts up. At first, you can clearly see the blades. The quicker the movement becomes, the more the contours are blurred, until it appears that there is a disk where the propeller blades used to be. Physics has also mathematically substantiated that quickly vibrating particles behave mechanically in a way quite similar to a solid body that fills out the space in which the particles move. You can easily comprehend how the movements of an object's particles react to the vibrations of the surrounding environment by placing a guitar, for example, next to a loudspeaker box as it reproduces music. You will hear a quiet tone if you hold your ear close to the strings. This means that they have begun to vibrate. However, such resonance phenomena is found not only in the field of acoustic energy.

Radiesthesia and Vibrations

In radiesthesia, the teaching of working with dowsing rods and pendulums, the influencing of a body's vibrations through external energy fields has long been used in order to find such things as water or ore concealed beneath the surface of the earth. When a person trained to use the pendulum or dowsing rod comes to a place above a water vein with this instrument, he or she can determine a very characteristic vibrational pattern. In this way, not only subtle energies can be proved, but also electromagnetic vibrations of all types. This is exactly where the matter begins to be interesting for us, since this book deals with perceiving subtle and electromagnetic forces through the human senses. Although a dowser or person using the pendulum still needs a "pointer" for the instrument body, he must at some point somehow have learned to register the fine vibrations of the surrounding environment with his senses and express them through a pendulum or divining rod. Let's take another look to see whether such an instrument is always necessary for this purpose.

The Body as a Pendulum

When I learned to work with the pendulum, I asked myself time and again how its vibrational pattern could come into existence. After I was quickly able to exclude a psychokinetic influence on the pendulum—moving it purely by mental power—the only other possibility was the unconscious activation of the smallest muscles in my body. Yet, how is the complicated movement of my muscles controlled while I hold the pendulum, and why isn't it strenuous for me to create a strong swinging motion, even if the pendulum is relatively heavy? What was it inside of me that reacted so sensitively to the energies of my surrounding environment and took shape in movements of the pendulum without my taking conscious notice of it? Time and again I attempted to understand these processes, but with-

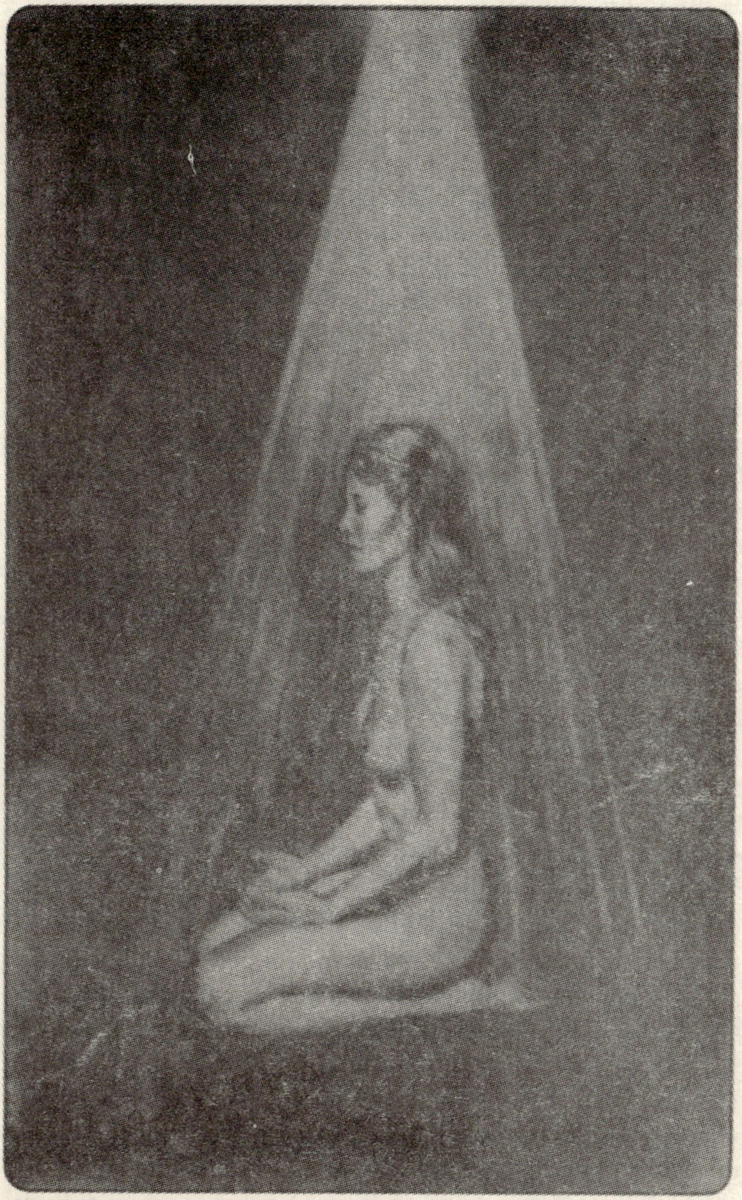

Meditating under a Reiki shower

out success at first. I still needed to have some experiences in other fields that were to give me the key to this puzzle. Some years later, I began with Tai Chi Chuan training and was astonished to discover that this had an important similarity with the phenomenon of the pendulum for me. My trainer insisted that I carry out all the movements of the preparatory special gymnastics and the complicated exercises of the Tai Chi form in a very relaxed and effortless way. At first I thought it would be impossible to practice like this—at least since I still distinctly remembered the sweat-producing training hours with other types of martial arts that I had learned, like judo and karate. However, after I had practiced Tai Chi for a longer period of time, I noticed after a few attempts that it was possible to practice without effort. But as soon as I noticed this, the great experience of being able to move as lightly as a feather was also over. In order to understand what this experience enabled me to do, I bought an abundance of books on Tai Chi. Over and over again, I read in them how effortless movement is the absolutely essential precondition for letting the Chi—the life energy—flow, and how the use of muscle power would immediately block it. However, none of the authors directly addressed how this effortlessness could be achieved. I didn't get any further here either, and long years passed before I became familiar with the many systems of personality development, accumulating many experiences with myself. One of them ultimately set the process of perception in motion that was necessary in order to put the puzzle together.

For some time I had been involved with meditation. In many painful hours I had experienced that it's not so easy to sit for a longer period of time with an upright pelvis and erect back. To also relax at the same time was impossible for me. But since I did want to learn to meditate, I came up with a trick. Using a method of the Second Reiki Degree, I created a so-called Reiki shower above the spot where I always meditated (or tried to ignore my aching back muscles). This is a stationary power field that lets the universal life energy flow to this spot for several hours. The first time I meditated under my energy shower, I had a strange experience: it was no longer difficult for me to sit with a straight back. To the contrary, I now had to make an effort if I wanted to round my back to the way in which it had felt more comfortable before. And after I sat relaxed in the meditation position for some time, my upper body started to sway

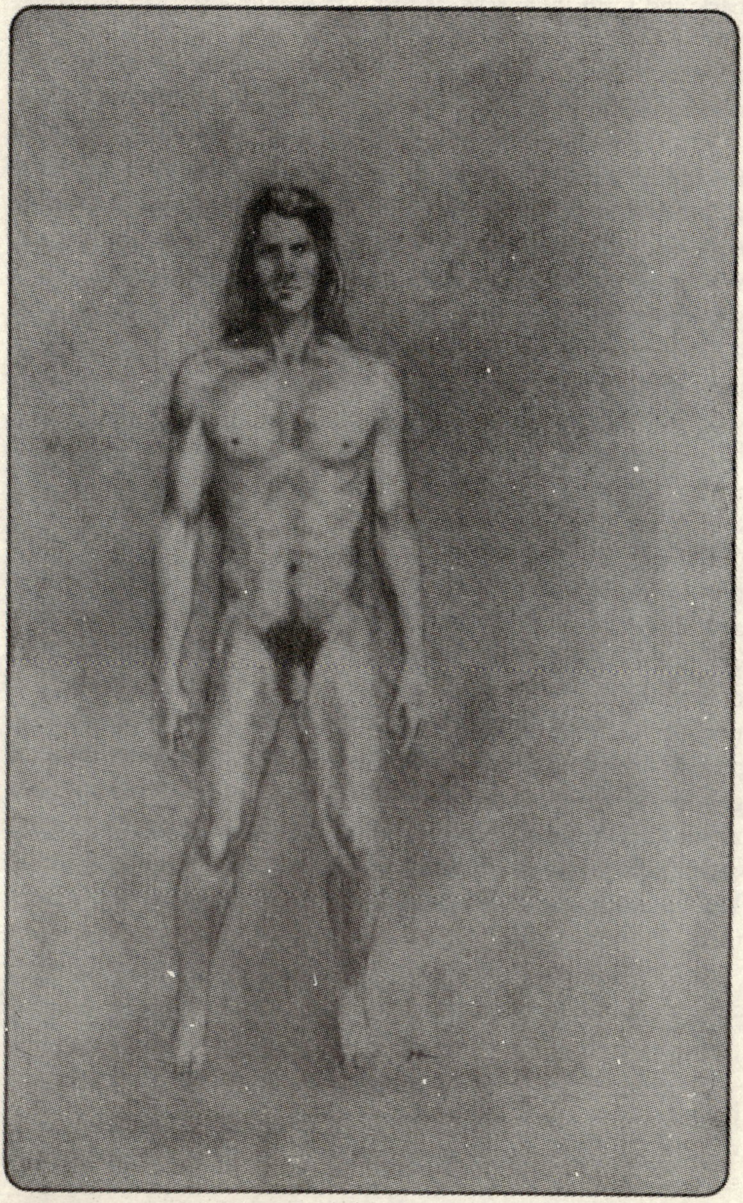

Basic posture, front view

back and forth in a circle, at first just slightly and then more distinctly. I was the pendulum! I didn't consciously produce this movement but it somehow happened to me. This time, the experience didn't stop once I became conscious of the process.

During the next few weeks, I was finally able to develop a well-founded system on the basis of this experience and my knowledge about the flow of bodily energies. This system explained my experiences with the pendulum and Tai Chi Chuan. Later, I worked out a system of physical exercises so that the body could also experience this understanding. These vibrational exercises that I developed are a simple possibility for anyone to experience his or her body as a pendulum, once again finding its individual rhythm and directly experiencing how the vibrations of the surrounding environment have an influence on the body. On the basis of my perceptions about the body's vibrational behavior and ability to resonate, and the practical application of this, anyone can immediately—and without any extra aids—determine whether a sleeping place is healthy for him, whether he has a harmonious energetic connection with another person, whether or not the microwave has an effect on him, and many other things. Oh yes, the preconditions for a direct view of the aura are also created with these exercises. But the exercises are not absolutely necessary for learning to read auras. Now that you probably can hardly wait to find out how this great stuff works, I'm going to skip over any further theories for the moment (for the rationalists: Don't worry! There will be enough explanations at the end of this chapter.) and introduce you to the resonance exercises. You can enter into direct contact with the world of energies with these.

The Resonance Exercises

Basic posture: This posture offers an optimal precondition for letting your body resonate. In order to work successfully with the resonance exercises, it's absolutely necessary to be able to correctly assume this posture.

Stand in an upright position with your legs about shoulder-width apart and the tips of your toes pointing somewhat inwards. Now bend your knees and shift your weight to the front so that your knees are above your toes. Your pelvis is upright, which means push your pelvis to the front. This automatically gives your body a bow-shaped posture. Your arms hang down relaxed, your head rests easily on your neck as if it was being pulled upwards by a string attached to the top of the head. When you have properly assumed this position, you can also relax the leg muscles since your body is now held in a balanced way. **(See "Basic posture" illustrations page 33 and 36.)**

Preparation Exercise 1

Perception Part A

It's useful to make a brief written note of your condition before and after the movement part. If you do this over a longer period of time, this will make an interesting journal on the development of your sensitivity. After several weeks, you will probably wonder about how "speechless" you were at the beginning of the exercise time in relation to your physical sense of perception. Writing things down will also help you in taking the perception exercise seriously and not just quickly passing over your sensations. Make it a point to note at least three sentences after every perception part. For this purpose, I bought myself a little silk-covered Chinese notebook in which I like to write.

Feel what's going on inside your body for a moment. First feel the feet, then the calves, up into the knees and thighs, then the lower abdomen and pelvic area, and then the upper abdomen and chest area, the shoulders, arms and hands, and finally the throat, jaw, and the head. This isn't a matter of perceiving anything in particular. Just focus on what's inside of you and register how you feel. Take the time to do this! Learning to sense what's going on inside yourself is very significant for allowing yourself to have subtle perceptions. The development of your sensitivity is more important than any other technique of energy work.

Movement Part

Now vigorously shake your hands, as if you wanted to shake off water. Allow your body to move along with this. Keep shaking until every region of the body is included in the movement. While doing this, your pelvis and head should remain straight but relaxed. When everything is shaking, continue for about 30 more seconds to determine whether you can permit yourself to let go of your body for a longer period of time.

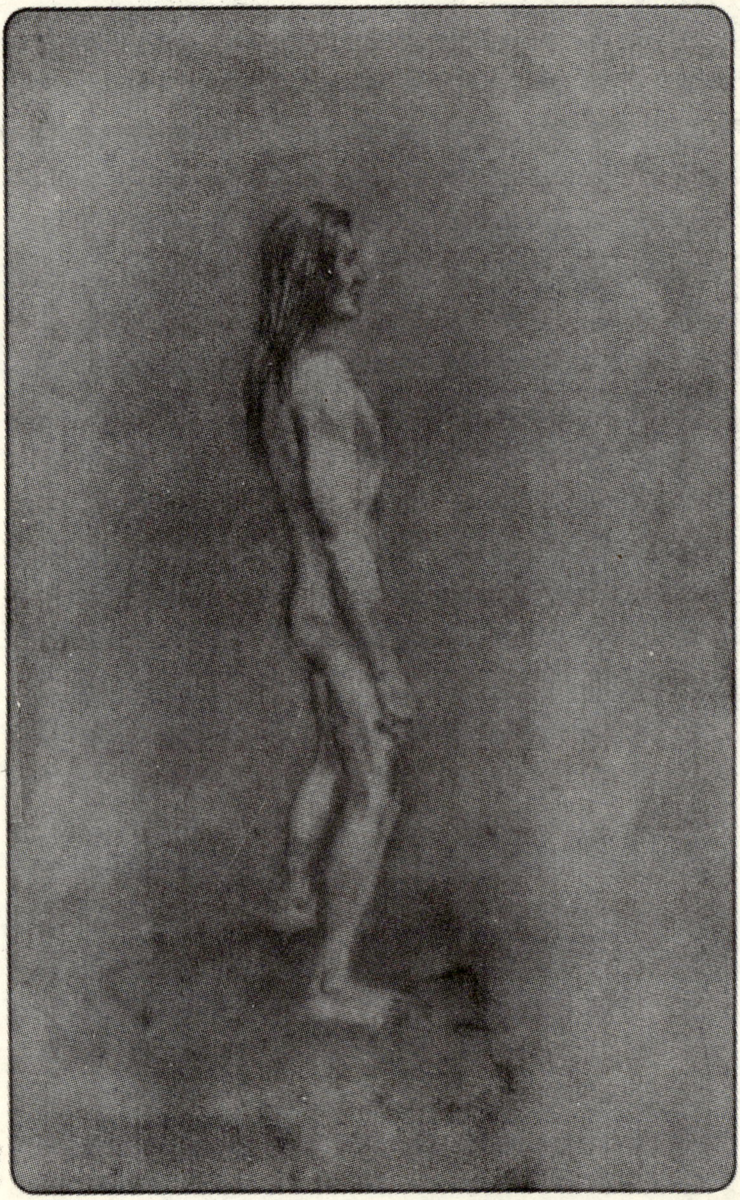

Basic posture, side view

Perception Part B
Now once again focus on your body, as described above in Perception Part A. Do you feel exactly like you did before the shaking exercise? Do you perceive any differences? If yes, where? Describe the difference in respect to the previous state for yourself.

When you have clearly(!) felt what's going on inside your present bodily state, then Preparation Exercise 1 is over.

Preparation Exercise 2
Perception Part A as in the Previous Exercise

Movement Part
Roll both shoulders alternately, as if you were doing the crawl stroke, without moving your arms. Let the movement be passed on to your entire body. Always keep the pelvis and the head upright while you do this. The arms and hands should be relaxed.

Do Perception Part B as in the previous exercise.

Preparation Exercise 3
Perception Part A
as in Preparation Exercise 1

Movement Part
Assume the basic posture and raise your arms while stretching them out, but without any stiffness, in front of your body as if you were holding a large ball. The right hand is to be held up and the left hand down while doing this. Now move your arms to the right and somewhat upward at the same time. Then let the lower arm come upward and the upper arm come downward, without pausing in the overall movement. Move both arms somewhat downward and then to the other side of your body. While doing this, lift them increasingly higher as they pass in front of your chest. When you have reached the top on the left side, let your arms change places once again and move them somewhat downward at the same time. From here, move them back up to the upper right side in an ascending line past your chest. The description may sound somewhat complicated, but it's basically quite simple: Your arms draw the figure of an infinity sign (an eight on its side) in front of your body (also see the illustration for Preparation Exercise 3). Let your entire body vibrate along with this exercise in a relaxed way when you do this move-

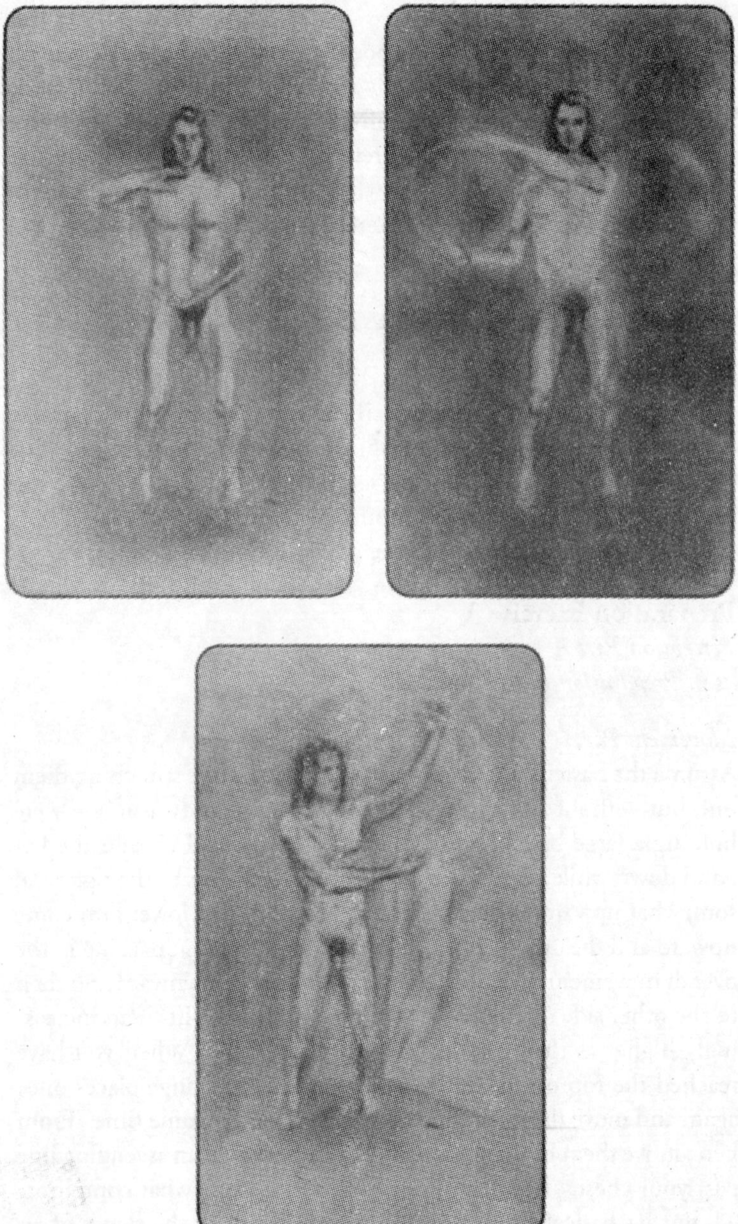

Preparation Exercise 3

ment. As described above, your pelvis and head remain upright and relaxed. Carry out this sequence of movements until you get totally caught in your own rhythm. The purpose of this exercise is to make it possible for you to clearly perceive your own personal vibration and let it fill your entire body.

The exercise has a direct activating effect on your heart chakra and indirectly strengthens your HARA. It will calm and relax you. And it will help you increase your overall feeling for your body.

The three preparatory exercises are only important for you until you can distinctly perceive the difference between tension and relaxation and have learned to quickly get into a posture that is relaxed and supports vibration. Later, you will only need it to become capable of vibrating and resonating when you are very tense.

Basic Exercise 1

Assume the basic posture and turn one shoulder as far as possible to the front, bend your upper body forward until it's almost horizontal with the floor, and let your arm hang down loosely. Place the other arm behind your back, with its palm facing away from the body. Now slowly walk through the room and let the arm in front hang down relaxed. Pay attention to how it swings, when it moves back and forth more easily, and when it becomes heavy. Stop every once in a while and wait to see what happens. In no case should you consciously influence the movements of your arm and use active muscle power! When you have practiced in this way for a few minutes, change to the other arm and do the exercise with it. When your arm and shoulder muscles are relaxed, your arm will make various circle, line, and ellipse figures, which you can also observe when working with a radiesthesic pendulum. If you are holding onto your arm at some place, it will only swing back and forth like an elephant's trunk. If this is the case, try to let go even more. If it doesn't even move while you're walking, then do the preparation exercises once again in order to learn to relax and let go. A frequent mistake that dooms the exercise to failure from the start is an improper pelvic posture. The pelvis must(!) be upright, meaning pushed forward. Become aware of the two different body postures by sitting on a chair and acting like you've swallowed a poker. But in no case should you have a hollow back. Now your pelvis is upright. Then let your body slump into what is usually felt to be a more comfortable

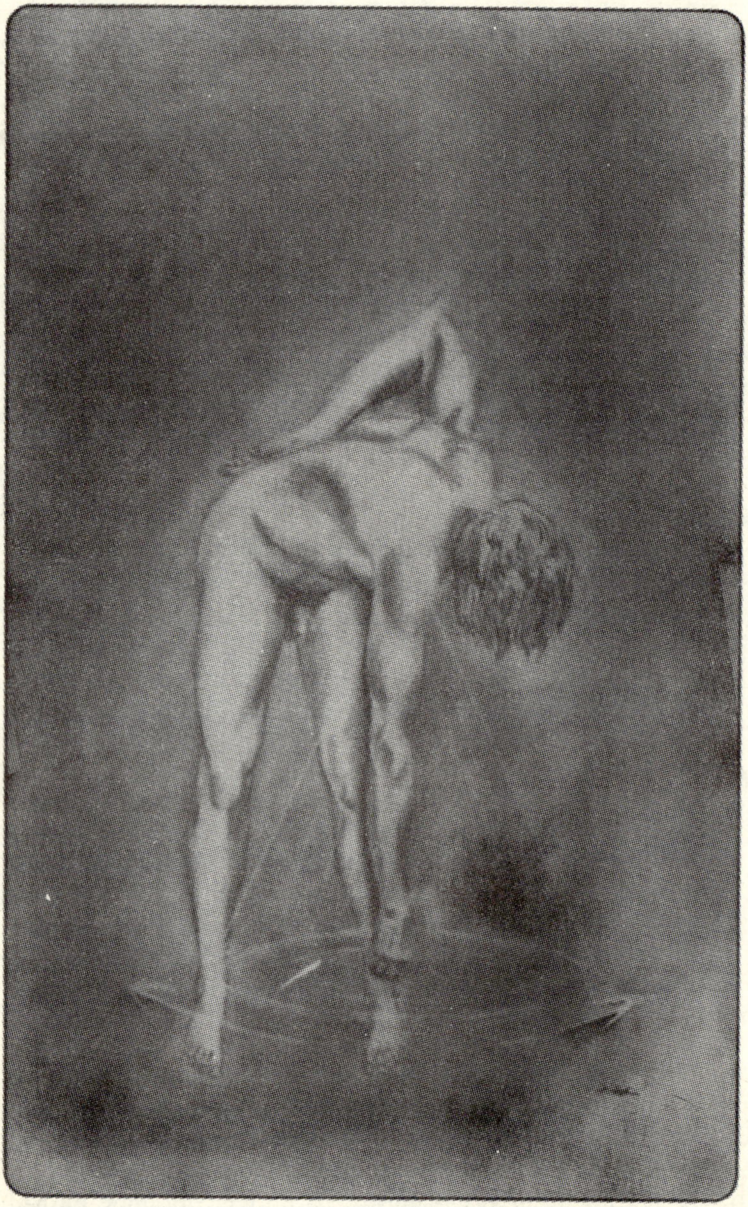

Basic Exercise 1

posture. Now your spinal column is no longer upright but pushed out to the back (rounded back).

Basic Exercise 1—Variation A

Once you've had some experience with this vibrational exercise, you can vary it by sitting on a chair and leaning your upper body to one side, but without turning it in this direction. Let your arm simply hang down on the slanted side and direct the palm of the hand on your other arm toward various places in your environment. Observe how your arm swings in each case. Repeat this exercise after a few minutes with the other side of the body and look at what differences and what similarities occur.

Basic Exercise 1—Variation B

Like Variation A. This time try out different places in the room that produce a strong swing in your pendulum arm when you hold the receiver arm in the respective direction. While doing this, straighten up your pelvis at one point and then slump down at another time. Observe how the swing of your pendulum arm changes. Then let your head hang forward at one time and straighten it up at another, as described in the basic posture. How does this change your ability to swing?

If you do this exercise correctly, your arm will immediately stop swinging when you bend your pelvis and immediately start moving again as soon as you straighten up your pelvis. It will do exactly the same thing when you let your head hang down and begin again when you hold your head erect as in the basic exercise.

Basic Exercise 1—Variation C

Do the pendulum exercise once again in a standing position. This time, slant your upper body just a little bit toward one side, similar to Variation A, and observe if you can also use your arm as a pendulum in this way. Also try out both pelvic positions and head positions here, and observe the effects on your ability to swing your arm.

Basic Exercise 2

While assuming basic position 1, stand at a spot where you had a strong swing during the previous exercises. Allow your upper body to begin to swing. If you have difficulties in letting go, then loosen up once again with the preparation exercises.

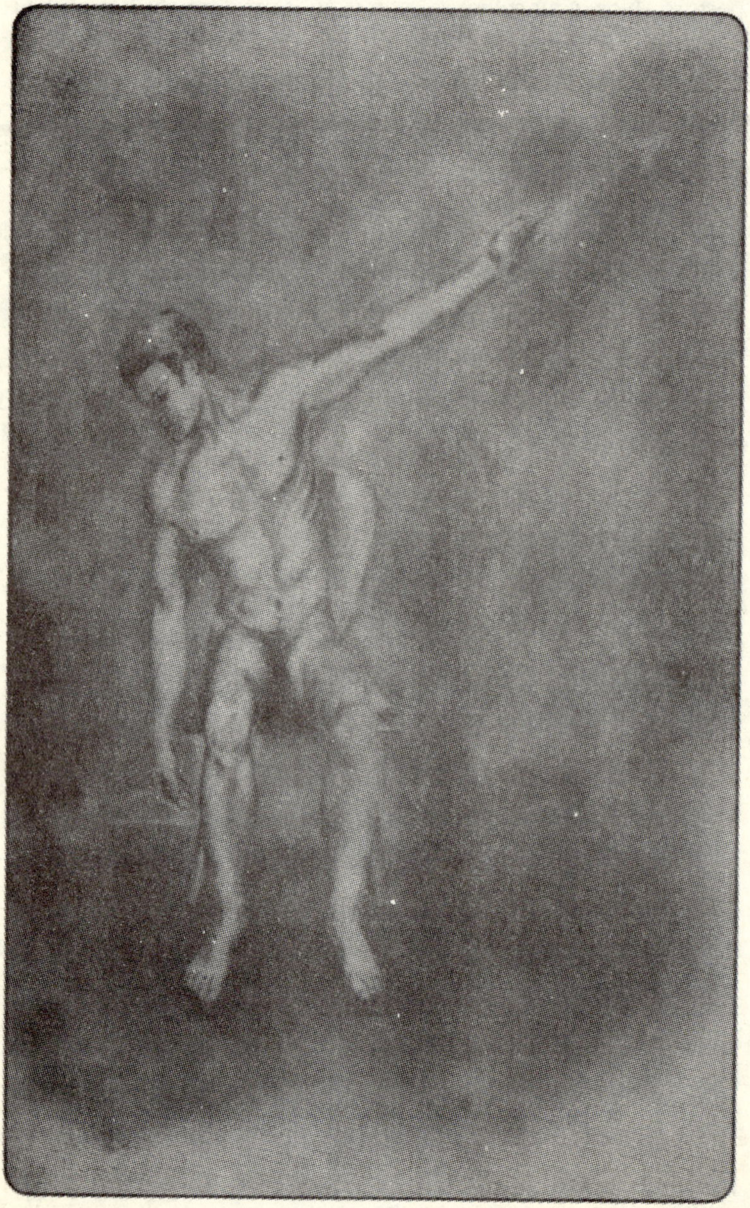

Basic Exercise 1–Variation A

Basic Exercise 2—Variation A

If you can cope well with the basic exercise 2, then you can also try out how your ability to swing changes with an upright pelvis and with a bent pelvis, as well as with both of the different head positions. Feel what's going on inside yourself in order to experience how your bodily perception changes in the various positions of the pelvis and head.

Basic Exercise 3

Sit on a chair with a solid surface and cross your arms in front of your chest. Place your feet one-and-a-half shoulder-widths apart with the soles flat on the floor. Straighten up your pelvis and your head. Allow your upper body to swing on the lumbar vertebrae. If you do well with this basic exercise, then also experiment with the various positions of the head and pelvis.

Basic Exercise 4

This exercise requires some preparation. It won't necessarily work out right away. Take your time in order to relax beforehand, and use the preparation exercise to train yourself in letting go. In no case should you put yourself under any pressure to succeed!

In the basic posture, stand at a spot with a strong vibration and permit your entire body to react. If you let go everywhere, you will soon be swinging from the ankle joints to the neck. While doing this, pay attention to a correct position of the pelvis and head. If you have difficulties, then do the preparation exercises one more time and then try it once again until your body clearly swings along with it.

Basic Exercise 4—Variation A

Experiment with both head and pelvis positions, paying attention to the differences so that you clearly develop your physical feeling for experiencing "what is capable of resonating" and "what isn't capable of resonating."

Basic Exercise 5

Like basic exercise 4. After you have let your entire body swing along, tap lightly with one finger on a spot, about three fingers below your navel in the center of your body. This is where, located somewhat within the body, you have your HARA, the mechanical and subtle center of your personality. Now again try to let your entire body swing along with the outer field. Pay attention to the correct position of the pelvis and head while you do this. Change a few times between the state of "attention in the HARA" and "attention not in the HARA," observing if there are differences in the feeling.

If you keep your attention in the HARA, your body will not longer swing back and forth, even if the pelvis and head are held correctly. If you take your attention away from the HARA, your body will once again swing back and forth.

Possible Effects on Resonance Exercises

If you practice the various fundamental techniques on a regular basis, you will once again achieve an important freedom of choice: you can now consciously switch between "resonating along" and "holding." In addition, you can also choose how you want to hold on. Since the exercises only work when you are truly relaxed, you can also use them as a highly effective form of relaxation exercises. If you practice them on a regular basis, your body will become increasingly capable of resonating and more flexible. The holistic ability to move will return. This means that you once again learn to feel and to move your body as a unity. Your movements will become lighter, more elegant, rhythmic, and powerful. Isolated body movements, in which just the arms change their position instead of including the entire body, for example, also mean isolated body perception and therefore an unnatural way of doing things that promotes tensions and blocks on the physical and mental levels. When you raise one arm, the weight of your body shifts. If you simply let the body react, it will adapt to the new situation through a slightly changed overall posture and can continue to be relaxed. Not permitting this automatic "level regulation" of your body requires a great deal of muscle work and promotes chronic tensions and anatomically unhealthy body postures with time.

Living Holistically—Moving Holistically

A holistic way of life begins with your body. Its posture is a mirror of your momentary mental attitude. But just as your mental area can influence your body, it's also possible to relax your mental attitude through the conscious acceptance of your physical reactions. Since this book follows a holistic concept, you can use both possibilities in order to learn how to perceive subtle energies and how to deal with them. You will find the same principle of automatic reaction to stimuli on the subtle energy level as well. If you simply permit it to happen and feel it, fantastic things will practically occur on their own and you will gain access to a great many useful abilities in this area.

Sense and Nonsense about So-Called Bad Posture

In order to more precisely explain the benefits of resonance exercises, we must back up a bit. You are sure to have heard more than once how very important it is for successful meditation to sit with an upright pelvis. In the various directions of physically oriented psychotherapy, great value is also placed on this as well. However, at the same time it is very painful and difficult for most people to sit in such a position for a longer period of time. They find it much more comfortable to sit in a slouched posture, even though this has been proven to be unhealthy. Why is this so? From your experience with resonace exercises, you know that your body can't swing along when the pelvis is bent. There is an explanation for this based on knowledge about the energetic structure of the human body.*

Three main conductor paths for life energy run in and next to the spinal column from the pelvis to the top of the head. In the special Indian language of Sanskrit, these three channels are called IDA, PINGALA, and SUSHUMNA. All six of the body's main chakras are connected with each other through these paths. The energy fields of the surrounding area, which are interesting for us within this context, are received by the second chakra (sexual chakra). This chakra is situated just above the pubic bone and distributes the energies on to the rest of the body from there through the three channels. These are then processed by the other chakras in accordance with their functions. The fifth chakra (self-expression chakra) is responsible for translating the energies it receives into physical expression (resonance), among other things. When you straighten up pelvis, the information from the second chakra can be conducted upward and translated into physical expression by the fifth chakra. If you bend your pelvis, the three conductive paths are obstructed in their function, and not enough information reaches upward to be transformed into intuitive body movements. Similar to a bent water hose, the energies now become congested in the lower back region. The situation is similar in the throat area. If you hold your head as

* You will find detailed explanations about the energy system and the chakras in Chapter 4. I will just go into the partial areas that are important for understanding the resonance exercises here.

if a string from the top was pulling it up to the sky, the head posture is optimal and promotes the energy flow in ida, pingala, and sushumna. If you tilt your head forward or backward, the conduction of stimulus is disrupted and no change of physical expression occurs.

But if this posture obstructs the normal and healthy functioning of the body, then why do so many people prefer to use it and find it more comfortable than the upright, healthier posture?

With the resonance exercises, you have had the experience that your body endeavors to be in harmony with the vibrations of the surrounding world. Similar to the above-mentioned raising of the arms and its resulting automatic change of the body's posture, which strives for a new equilibrium, this feedback mechanism also functions on the level of subtle energy. This is quite practical since much more information flows in this way. Dangers and advantageous situations can be more easily and quickly recognized. Energetic communication with other beings helps us to be accepted by them. And environmental energies can be used as sources of energy when the body adapts to the vibrations that support it in its respective movements with their rhythm. At the same time, this precludes a waste of energy since the energetic equilibrium of the body remains intact. Community makes us strong, and not just in the emotional sense.

However, in our current age we are constantly surrounded by hundreds of different sources of vibrations such as electrical power lines and devices, gatherings of people, earth emanations, functional radio stretches, television and radio waves, satellite signs, advertizing billboards, newspapers, television films, books, and so on and so forth. Many of these are very strong and contain an enormous amount of information. It's impossible for our body to adapt to this great number of rhythms and process them. In addition, particularly in heavily populated areas, the energy fields change constantly. This subjects the body's organs, which are occupied with the translation and evaluation of the absorbed stimuli, to a tremendous state of continuous stress. Even when we sleep, we are for the most part helplessly at the mercy of the fields from radio alarm clocks, electrical facilities, and radio signals.

If the body were to attempt to remain completely receptive and express all the energies that flow into it, it would quickly break down because of the overload. In this difficult situation, our wise body consciousness simply pulls the most accessible emergency brake and reduces the further conduction of stimuli to the absolutely necessary minimum (bent pelvis, tilted head), which obstructs the main conductive system in and along the spinal column in its function. The frequently criticized bad posture of human beings living in modern civilization is then nothing more than a drastic self-help measure by the body to ensure its survival and ability to function in the here and now—even at the price of a long-term damage to its functional capacity. This is why simply telling someone to change his or her posture (stand up straight!) or training the muscles to make an upright posture possible (body-building, etc.) can't produce any kind of true success. If the body would permit a relaxed and vibrationally open upright posture during constant overstimulation, under certain circumstances this would be like suicide; in any case, it would constantly overload a great portion of its reaction possibilities.

Now pay attention to whether it's easy for you sit with a straight pelvis and head. If the place is energetically completely neutral (rare) or if it has just a few, balanced energies, then (after a brief transition period) it won't be a problem for you—and you may even like it—to sit up straight. Then look for another place that has an imbalanced energetic situation and repeat the exercise there. It will at least be much more difficult for you to sit up straight. Also try out this exercise in your home. Perhaps you will even find a place in your home that proves to have quite balanced energies. A tip: with the incense (frankincense, for example) available at specialized esoteric stores, you can harmonize at least many of the energy impressions that don't constantly renew themselves. If you have the Second Reiki Degree, you can use a Reiki shower in a simple way to create a meditation place for yourself in your favorite spot of your home. (Also see the chapter on the Second Reiki Degree in my book *Reiki—Way of the Heart.*) If you have Bach Flowers, you can also try using a few drops of the Rescue Remedy before a mediation session. The Rescue Remedy drops briefly have an effect similar to a strong activation of the HARA. The experience that energetically balanced places benefit mediation and opening up to inner perceptions has been a familiar one since ancient times. This knowledge was still taken into express consideration when building churches and monasteries until about one-hundred years ago. Adepts of a great variety of confessions such as yogis, shamans, Christian mystics, and Taoist masters preferred to retreat to such balanced places because this enabled them to develop their perceptive abilities without obstruction through external influences.

Activating the Hara to Set Energetic Limits

Bent body posture isn't the only method for protecting ourselves from undesired stimuli. As you have learned from the resonance exercises, directing your attention to your HARA also has a similar effect, even if your posture remains upright while doing so. However, this way of setting limits is much healthier and even promotes your development. Directing your attention to your HARA connects your second chakra with your third chakra so that the incoming energies are sent directly on to the "main transformer"—the solar plexus chakra—to be transformed and stored for later purposeful use. The more energies that flow in you now, the better. They will all be integrated into your energy system and thereby strengthen you. So directing your attention to the HARA is a something that's really great. In order to truly make use of the incoming vibrations in this harmonious way, you will need some practice. At the beginning you will most likely actually integrate about 3–5% of the energy flowing to you. But even this amount, which may appear to be quite minor to you, will very much relieve your energy system and provide it with a great deal of fresh energy under certain circumstances. Practice with your HARA on a regular basis and check your progress time and again.

Practical Applications of Strengthening the Hara

Even in the ancient Asian methods of meditation, much value is placed on directing the attention to this region because of the reasons mentioned above. A great many exercises have been developed in order to check the progress of the practitioner and train the practical application of these energies. I would like to introduce one of these now so that you can experience the practical use of this form of energy work. You need a partner to do it.

Stand facing each other with about half a meter between you. Hold one arm at stomach level with the back of the hand facing away from you at a distance of about 30 cm. With his stronger hand, your partner now takes hold of your wrist. Then tell him to "hold!" and now try to push him away from you with the muscle power of your arm. Even with a great deal of effort, you probably won't have

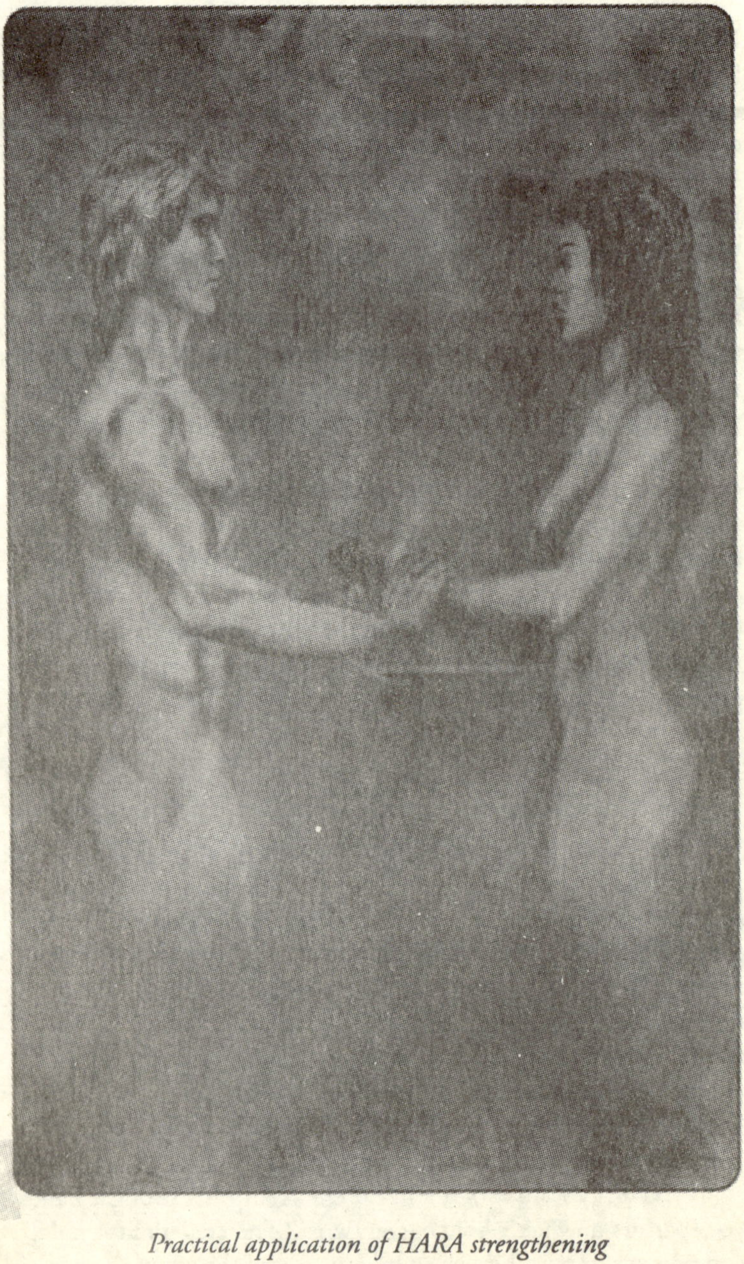

Practical application of HARA strengthening

much success in doing this. Now close your eyes for a moment and direct your attention to your HARA. Feel how an increasing amount of energy collects there. When you clearly perceive this strength, say "hold!" again. Let the energy from your abdominal area shoot into your arm and let it be carried forward by the energy. If you do the exercise correctly, your partner will at least clearly notice the difference. He will usually be downright shoved away by it.

Unfortunately, there's not enough space here to list further exercises of this type since this present book is primarily concerned with once again opening up to subtle, energetic perception. If you are interested in this form of energy work, please refer to the commented bibliography at the end of the book. Two excellent books by the Japanese Ki master Koichi Tohei are listed, from which you can learn more about the Ki exercises, their technical name. At the moment it's just important that you learn to work a bit with your HARA so that your body consciousness doesn't have to constantly pull the emergency brake of "round your back" and "bend your neck." Through HARA work, you can also safely subject yourself to stronger energetic influences. Then you will never drift like a rudderless boat in the storm but be guided by your reliable helmsman (HARA) with a sail (second chakra) and rudder (third chakra), applying the power of the environment's energies for your own well-being.

The Heart Chakra and Subtle Perceptions

But this isn't all that you can receive in the way of lovely gifts when you make use of the vibrational theory and the vibrational exercises. You may remember the Preparation Exercise 3 described above. It has a very important function that I must explain so that you have some absolutely necessary knowledge about the development of your energy system. One specific benefit of this exercise is that it enables you to harmoniously and quickly develop your heart chakra. And this chakra is associated with the organ in your body that can ultimately give you access to energies stored in your third chakra (solar plexus center), which are then available for your use. Without the development of your heart chakra, there's no way for you to have a deeper insight into auras. So let's take a closer look at this area in order to become more familiar with its function.

Everything in this world has a vibration. Even human beings. You've already taken a closer look at how our vibrations are changed through external influences. With the Preparation Exercise 3, you have also experienced a possibility of getting back into contact with your own rhythm. But where does your personal vibration come from?

There is a "rhythm generator" within the human body that is in operation for an entire lifetime. If it stops, the affected person will die within a short time. This generator is the heart. It is the only muscle in the body that has its own time-giver, meaning that it isn't causally controlled by the brain. This time-giver is divided into three autonomous nerve centers: the sinoatrial node of the upper heart region in the area of the superior vena cava, which is also called the heart's pacemaker and dictates the basic rhythm of 60–80 beats for an adult. Its impulses are directed through the vestibular musculature of the heart's right side to the atrioventicular node, the second portion of the "rhythm generator," which is located in the lower portion of the right vestibule. From there, the impulses flow to the so-called atrioventricular bundle, the third nerve node of this vibration generator, which is located approximately beneath the artioventricular node.

Although these three centers form a functional unit, they are also capable of working on their own. If the sinoatrial node stops working for some reason, the artrioventricular node takes over its timing-keeping function. However, its frequency of 40–60 beats/minute isn't as high as that of that sinoatrial node. If this center also quits working, the atrioventricular bundle tries to take over its task. But its heartbeat frequency of 30–40 beats/minute is even lower. Since only the sinoatrial node with its relatively high number of beats can provide smooth functioning of the heart-circulatory system, when it ceases to work, a mechanical time-giver is installed to guarantee a sufficiently high beat frequency with its electrical impulses. Although the stimuli-conduction system of the heart can be influenced from the outside through the sympathetic nerve and the vagus nerve within certain limits, the fundamental control over the heart's own time-giver cannot be replaced by any other organ of the body. The basic rhythm of your heart is your own personal rhythm. It can be felt everywhere in your body as a pulsation. The blood with its vessels serves as the heart's ambassador. It attempts to pass on the vibration of love to all the cells of the body and thereby maintain contact with the source of life, which some people call God.

If the muscles in some regions of the body are cramped because the respective person is afraid of being lively and doesn't want to feel himself here, the pulse beat to the areas is passed on either in a subdued way or not at all. Less blood flows to the cramped areas as well. Under these conditions, metabolic waste products can easily become deposited and promote all types of diseases. The vibration of the heart brings life, detachment from this rhythm brings sickness and death.

The Positive Effects of Heart Vibrations

When a baby hears its mother's heartbeat, which it still recognizes from the time before birth, it calms down and feels safe and secure. Music with this beat frequency, which corresponds to the heartbeat, is used by such methods as "Superlearning" according to Professor Lozanov in order to tremendously increase people's ability to learn and keep them in a pleasantly relaxed, receptive state while doing so. If you learn to move to the beat of your heart, which occurs automatically when you do something like Preparatory Exercise 3, you will be more relaxed, powerful, and flexible in your movements since you work with, instead of against, the vibration of love within yourself. To more easily understand this, imagine that you are trying to dance a waltz at a party while the band plays a tango. Difficult, isn't it? But if you also dance the tango to the tango rhythm, it will be a lot of fun. By accepting your personal vibration, you will also quite automatically move in a holistic way since the rhythm is present within your entire body. This type of movement reduces tensions of all types with time and prevents new ones from occurring. This leads to an improved metabolism, reduces waste materials, and over a longer period of time thereby decreases the tendency to become sick.

People still were aware of these effects of moving in the natural rhythm several decades ago. For example, the farm workers threshed the straw and sang songs with such a time frequency while they did so. Work in traditional handicraft occupations was accompanied by singing that set the corresponding rhythm, and in the military there is an ancient tradition of rhythmic singing on long marches since soldiers don't get tired as easily and it helps keep them in a good mood.

Preparatory Exercise 3 should help you bring natural momentum back into your life and get away from the arrhythmical hectic movement patterns of our age. It's naturally not enough for you to carry out this exercise for 10 minutes once a day. The goal of this vibrational exercise is for you to do the greatest portion of your daily activities in your own personal rhythm again. In this way, you will achieve much more for yourself than through years of daily practice isolated from your everyday life. Now you may ask how you should do all your activities of the day at one speed? The solution is quite simple: As in overtone singing, harmonically higher frequencies can result from a basic tone. But you don't need to know anything about music theory in order to make use of this principle. Let go of your body—you already know how to do it. If you let go, everything will start working harmoniously on its own after a short period of transition. *Don't push the river—it flows by itself...!*

Here's one last comment about the function of the heart chakra in relation to perceiving subtle energies. I spoke about the three autonomous time-givers of the heart above, the sinoatrial node, the artrioventricular node, and the atrioventricular bundle. These three nerve centers are connected with three of the subtle bodies*. The sinoatrial node is associated with the mental body here, the emotional body is connected to the artrioventricular node, and the etheric body with the atrioventricular bundle. In this respect, the heart is ultimately a reception station for the energetic vibrations of our subtle bodies. It is the chakra of unity, in which the life streams of the material and the subtle world unite and an exchange takes place. If I accept this function of my heart chakra and open my body for the vibration of love that emanates from it, I participate at the same time in the constant stream of information from the subtle world that flows to me with the heart vibrations. The ability to see auras, be clairvoyant and clairsentient, emotiopathy, and many other subtle senses are automatically awakened if you permit yourself to once again live in the rhythm of love.

You have had your first experiences with the direct perception of subtle energies in this chapter and learned something about the background of your subtle senses. Once you have carefully carried out the exercises, you should be prepared for the next chapter. This deals with the practical foundation for seeing auras.

---

* For a more detailed explanation of the subtle bodies, see Chapter 4.

Chapter 3

Practice: The First Steps to Reading the Aura

So, now it's time to start seeing auras! If you have carefully done the exercises in the last chapter, you can now already perceive quite a bit in the subtle area. Now you can go on to learning how to see energetic phenomenon. However, before you continue to read, please make one thing clear to yourself: It's not enough to read a book in order to learn to see and interpret the aura in some way. You need personal experiences. So it's very important that you do the exercises described in this chapter in a careful way and on a regular basis, until they have fulfilled their function for you. Yes, and that's all you need as a prerequisite for starting with clairvoyance.

What—you think that can't be enough? You're not yet highly developed, still eat meat, don't meditate every day, and sometimes swear like a fishwife? Well, these things have hardly obstructed your other five senses up to now, or have they? So go ahead—trust yourself and let's try this out together.

Your first exercise should help you open up to subtle perceptions. This isn't a matter of developing new senses but learning to use those that you have had since birth.

Directing Your Attention to the Subtle Senses

When you are at a concert where the music very much appeals to you, you listen quite precisely to it. You focus your attention on the music. If you like it very much, you will be all wrapped up in it. Your entire perceptive ability is then directed into one sensory organ. Without any intentions, you devote yourself to the experience of listening. But if you were to have an animated conversation with a friend during the concert, you would hear little of the music. Perhaps the noise level would even bother you. The same thing applies to seeing auras. Here as well, your attentiveness is decisive for the quality and depth of your perception. Directing attention does not mean concentration. Both of these processes even produce opposite results. If you concentrate, you willfully attempt to limit your sensory perceptions by having your intellect make a selection among the sensory stimuli that you take in. Concentration is never without intention. It always excludes certain perceptions that are undesirable at the moment. But since you don't even know what sort of impressions are coming at you before you perceive something, a great deal of important information can be suppressed in this manner. Let's go back to the example of the concert: Within this context, concentration means that you listen to the music with the intention of just paying attention to the first violin. Here directing your attention means letting yourself fall into the listening experience—being in a state of listening.

Concentration is exertion. But every act of holding on obstructs your unconscious mind in the communication with your consciousness. Directing attention means letting go, opening up for feeling the flowing energy. This is why in the old traditions of spiritual training so much value is placed on letting go. Concentration is essentially a method of making a preliminary selection of sensory impressions. Someone who concentrates assumes that in a certain situation he will know exactly what perceptions are worth being admitted. However, since the world can never be comprehended in a holistic way by the intellect, which is what directs concentration, in most cases it's impossible for the respective person to permit the perceptions important in the holistic sense by concentrating. Sometimes, this way of dealing with the world is necessary and proper. However, this is much more seldom than we believe. Directing attention is one method of consciously opening up to the perception of a situation. Instead of switching on a filter from the very start, the body consciousness is given the opportunity of making a selection. In the process, you can watch it or "feel it" and calmly think about what comes to you through your consciousness, your intellect. Since your body has access to the level of unity through your heart, it will always adapt to the most important perceptions for you in the holistic sense. Just learn to trust it once again! For those interested in the Asian way of thinking: This way of approaching the senses by directing the attention without concentration is called WU WEI, acting by not acting, in the Taoist philosophy. Many meditative and practical exercises of this tradition of initiation are only possible and useful through WU WEI.

How can you now achieve this direction of attention in a simple way?

Basic Exercises for Learning to See the Aura

Please take note: All these exercises should be done as often as possible in the same room, at the same spot. Then it will be easier for you to open up to learning on the basis of your subconscious mind. In addition, with time this place will have its own quality of promoting development, which also makes activities like meditation easier. After a longer period of time, a type of personal power place will be created if the preconditions for it are good.

By the way, if you do the following exercises on a regular basis and in a serious way, they will initiate self-healing reactions on all levels. So don't become frightened if you can feel the symptoms of old health disorders for a few days, if your perspiration or stool smells differently, if you are in a bad mood for a while, or if feelings come up within you that you hadn't discovered within yourself up to now. You may be experiencing detoxification reactions. The exercises can't harm you if you carry them out as described.

There is one important exception to this: Should you be in psychiatric or psychological treatment, then please discuss with the therapist treating you whether exercises 1 and 2 are suitable for you at this time. This precautionary measure is sometimes necessary because in certain types of serious psychological disorders an intensified opening of the physical perception without therapeutic accompaniment can lead to a change for the worse in the patient's well-being. Should you be in such a situation at the moment, you can also ask your therapist whether the two of you could perhaps do the exercises together for a while, at least until it's certain that you can cope with them. Through their healing power, they can make a substantial contribution to your recovery, and at the same time you are preparing yourself for the further exercises for learning to see auras.

Exercise 1

Preparation: Set an alarm clock or an egg timer (if possible, a mechanical one because of the electromagnetic field that radiates from electrically operated devices, or at a distance of at least 2 meters so that the field doesn't disturb the ritual) so that it rings after 3 minutes. Then you can let go of your appointments and not be disturbed in opening up to the following exercise. The clock should face away from you. Turn down your telephone and doorbell. If necessary, put a "DON'T DISTURB" sign on the door of your room. It's best to make one that will last for a longer period of time since you will need it for almost every exercise. Look for a quiet spot. You shouldn't use music and incense for this exercise. If you want to learn to feel within yourself, you must eliminate as many diversions as you can and keep them away from you.

Course of exercise: Sit down or lay down comfortably, close your eyes and pay attention to the flow of your breath. Once you have become calm, ask your Inner Child to help you in the following exercise. Tell it that you would like it to give you a clear sign when it no longer wants to practice, then promise to listen to this sign and end the exercise. Keep your promise! In return, ask it to help you do the exercises on a regular basis and learn them quickly and effortlessly. Then lightly(!) tap on the place about three fingers below your navel at the center of your body with a fingertip. Perceive the sensation of touch and remain there with your attention. At this place, one to two fingers beneath the skin, is where your HARA is located. When you direct your perception to this point by paying attention to the light touch, you will balance your energy system: This tends to relax your musculature and calms down your "thinking apparatus." If you notice that you are beginning to think about things or that your attention is wandering to other perceptions, then tap on your HARA again and feel what's going on there.

Stay with this exercise until the alarm clock rings. Do this little meditation every day for a week; if you like, you can also do it twice a day. During the next weeks, increase the length of the exercise to five minutes, then to ten minutes in the following week. And don't worry: you don't need to do this meditation until the end of your days, even though it can have a great many effects for you that promote your health and development if you make it a part of your daily routine. The purpose of this exercise for learning to see the

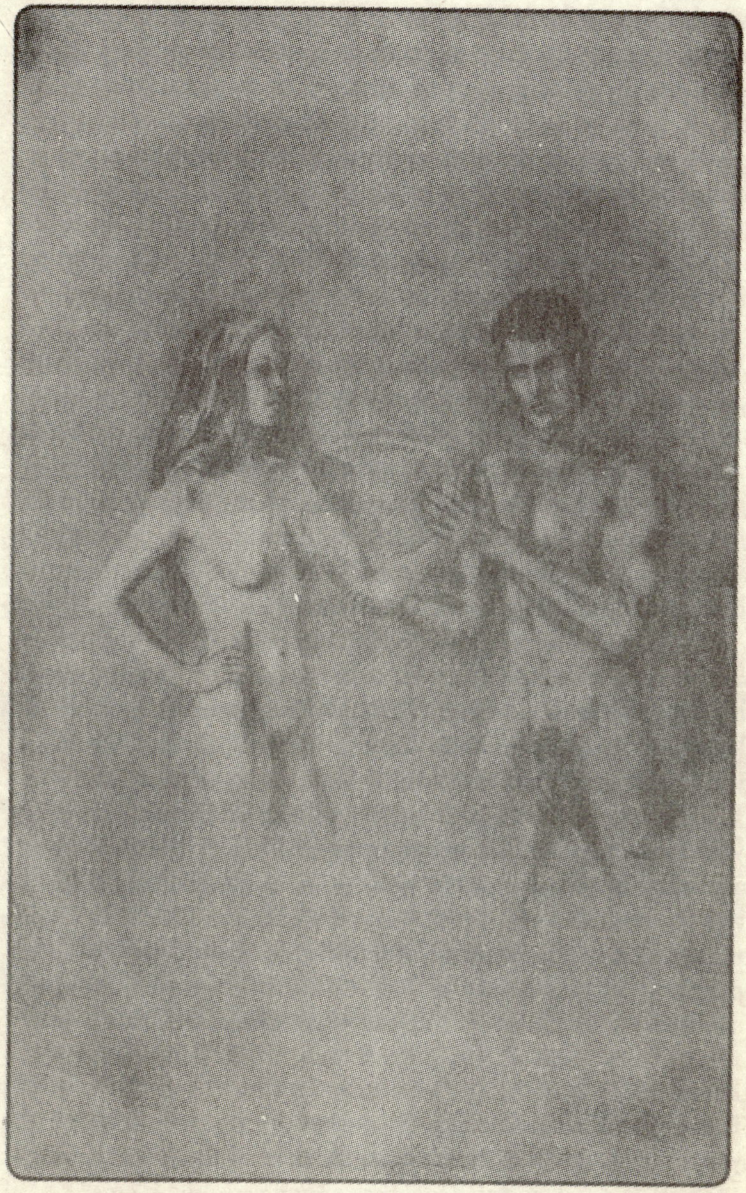

"The Iron Arm"

aura is just that you succeed in quickly, safely, and simply relaxing yourself on the physical and mental level, as well as being able to center yourself. Even if you are experienced in other relaxation exercises, you should carry out this exercise for a number of weeks since this initiates other processes of increasing consciousness that you may have been familiar with up to now. The following exercises are built on these processes.

There is a simple test to determine to what extent you have learned to correctly do the HARA meditation: This partner exercise comes from AIKIDO with KI, which has been developed by the Japanese master Koichi Tohei (also see bibliography). It's called the "Iron Arm." (See illustration on page 59) To do this, stand in a relaxed position, the feet about shoulder-width apart. Now lift your right arm and bend it to about 45 degrees. Your partner stands next to you and holds your elbow joint with one hand and your wrist with the other. Then let him press your lower arm toward your body and resist this with your muscle power in order to get a feeling for your strength and his (also see illustration "The Iron Arm" with respect to body posture and course of the exercise.

In preparation for the second part of the test, now direct your attention to your HARA. If you have the feeling of clearly perceiving it, give your friend a sign. Now he should once again press your lower arm toward your body. Don't tense your muscles! Just be in your HARA and hold your arm with the energy of your center.

If you are centered, your partner will have difficulty in moving your lower arm. If you are completely in your HARA with your attention, he won't be able to move your arm despite all his efforts and you won't have to use any muscle power to hold it. Carry out this test every few weeks in order to objectively determine your progress. When you have worked with the first exercise for about one week, you can also start doing the next one at the same time.

Exercise 2:

Preparation: As described under exercise 1. Also take a mirror with you to your place of practice. A cosmetic mirror (that doesn't enlarge!) of about 15 cm diameter is adequate. But it can also be larger.

Course of exercise and explanation: Directly before the exercise, look at your face in the mirror. Don't pay any attention to skin blemishes, wrinkles, or the color of your complexion. Look at yourself in the same way that you look at a person in the moment that you fall in love with him or her. You will immediately notice when you look the "right" way. At that moment, you will feel a sensation of tingling or warmth in the area of your heart. This is the heart look. You will need it time and again when you read auras. With the heart look, you can use the ability of your heart chakra for receiving subtle vibrations and are protected against unpleasant influences at the same time. It is a well-known phenomenon that people who, for example, use the pendulum a great deal or are good at seeing auras are also easily influenced by vibrations that are inharmonious for them. The effects of this can range from tiredness and exhaustion to sudden, unmotivated emotional outbursts. Dowsers who frequently find places with cancer-promoting vibrations often become ill themselves after a number of years if they don't know how to protect themselves. Since you open yourself for a great many different vibrations when you learn to see auras (otherwise you couldn't even perceive them), it is very important for you to learn to protect yourself. An important basic protection is the contract with yourself (see end of Chapter 1), which you have hopefully entered into by now. Among other things, through this promise, you put yourself under the protection of the powers of light and love* on a very deep personal level. However, the levels closer to your conscious mind are not protected extensively enough by this (perhaps you're starting to notice that I'm a fan of safety first—my practical experiences, which haven't always been pleasant, have made me this way ...).

The next protection is given to you with exercise 1. When you have learned to be at your center with your consciousness, you can no longer be thrown off balance as easily. Put in less metaphoric terms: Your aura is much stronger and your energetic detoxification system functions somewhat better when your attention is in your HARA. The last protection is "heart seeing." The subtle levels can be perceived quite well through all the chakras. But most of them become overloaded with time if you don't constantly do exercises that normalize them, which are relatively difficult to

---

* Even if you are already a member of the White Brotherhood or similar societies, this doesn't make this contract superfluous! Its effect extends very deep into your soul and opens you up for the development of uncompromising love.

learn. For the exercises to be effective, they must be individually adapted by an experienced master and modified time and again during the student's development. This is why my system is built on the activation of the heart chakra, the safest window to the subtle world for "normal mortals." This way, you perceive the energies with the eyes of love, of unity. This automatically neutralizes harmful impulses for you and/or lets you notice quickly, with certainty and in due time when inharmonious impressions flow into you that you can't process at the moment so that you can get out of the perceptive channel. Then the heart chakra is your personal "body guard." The thymus gland, which is associated with it, is also an important organ of the body's own immune system for protecting against pathogens of all sorts. If you love yourself, you also protect yourself against dangers ... If you have the feeling that you can't deal with a perception, direct your attention—as you have learned—to your HARA. This will make you strong and safe. You should in any case let some time pass (2–3 hours) before you take a closer look at the source of the disruptive perceptions on the subtle level. Practice this switching from seeing with the heart to HARA meditation time and again until you can master it with certainty at any time.

Seeing with the heart will also help you from the beginning to not let your personal prejudices flow into the subtle perception of another individual. In addition, with this type of seeing you are truly open to be completely with the other person and are therefore not as easily distracted: You know how this is with you when you're in love. When you have learned to see with the heart, you will develop the ability to perceive God in the other person....Practice this seeing with the heart every day for 3 minutes for one week (don't forget to set the alarm!), and then for 5 minutes a day the next week, and 10 minutes a day the week after. Once you have truly mastered seeing with the heart and the HARA meditation during the practice time, try them both out in your everyday life. But first just with yourself! When you go to the movies or take the subway, you can use the opportunity to briefly direct your attention to your HARA. Or close your eyes for a moment and observe your face in front of your inner eyes with the heart look. An expansion of Exercise 2 that you can try out when you have a good mastery of the first part is looking at your entire body in the mirror and then observing it in front of your inner eyes. Make it easy on yourself and first go through one body region at a time. For example, take a look at your right arm and then your left arm. Continue with your chest, your abdomen, etc. If you succeed in doing this, then look at increasingly larger areas of your body with the heart look through your inner eyes until you can visualize all of it without any difficulties, without going off at a tangent.

You should be totally secure in doing Exercises 1 and 2 before you continue. They are the foundation upon which the other exercises are built.

Exercise 3:

Preparation: Make a number of doubly enlarged copies of the illustration for Exercise 3 on page 64 (sketch of a human body with the front and back view) and place these pages together with a soft pencil within reaching distance. Do the rest of the preparation as in Exercise 1.

Course of exercise: Do the HARA meditation for three to five minutes. Then take a look at yourself with your inner eyes by seeing with your heart, as you have learned, and choose a certain region of your body that you would like to examine more closely such as your abdomen. Now formulate the wish in your mind to see the areas of congested, stuck energy covered with black. Pay attention to how the picture changes. Don't spend much time on interpreting and thinking (very important!) about what exactly your perception may represent. Instead, immediately draw what you have seen on one of the copied pages. Trust yourself and what you see. If you think you don't see anything, there is another approach. Ask yourself, "What would it be like if I could see something?" End the exercise when the time is up and the alarm clock rings.

It's important to start slowly with this since your subconscious mind needs time to process and integrate the new impressions. You will usually notice that this is too much for you if you develop an aversion to the sessions and try to find excuses so that you don't have to do them. Then allow yourself a break. Don't try to keep practicing despite your aversion but give yourself time to integrate the experiences you have collected up to now. Start practicing again when you sense that you have become curious about it or you have a desire

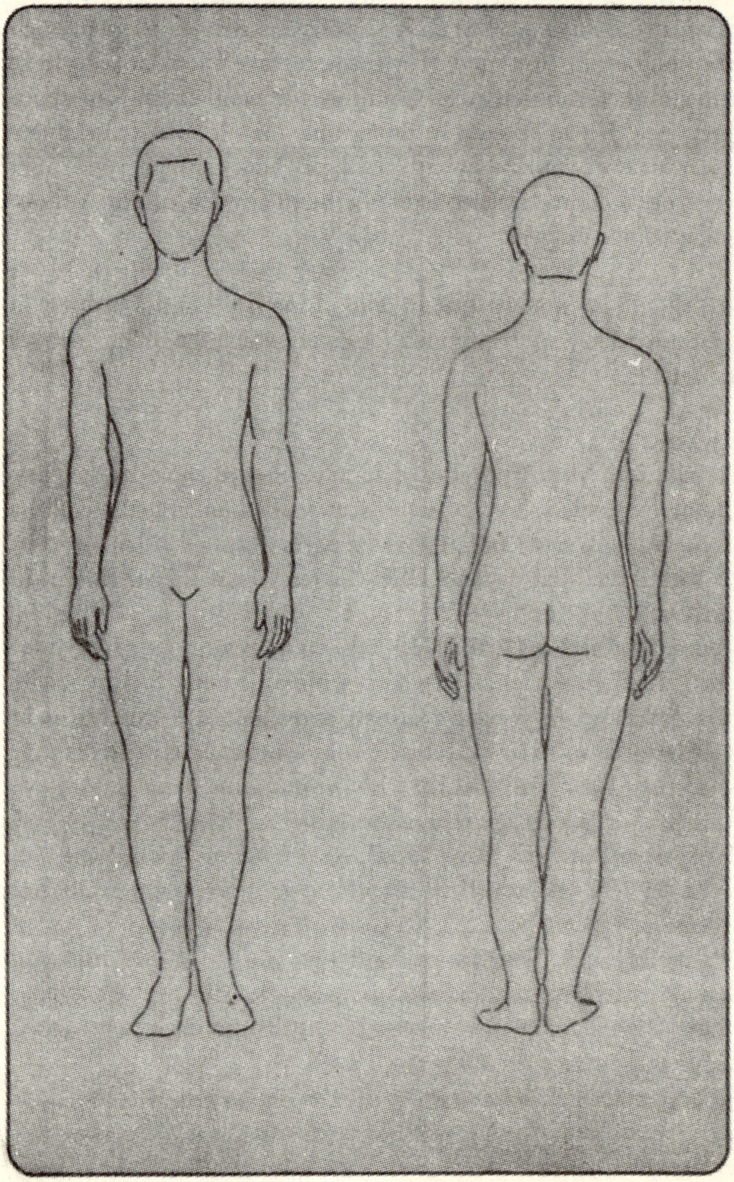

to do it again. As in the first two exercises, work 3 minutes a day on this type of inner vision for one week, then 5 minutes the next week, and 10 minutes the following week. At the conclusion of each session, do the HARA meditation for a moment in order to center yourself for everyday life.

Don't be afraid when you discover blocks within yourself, which will be the case with great probability. Each us has them. This usually doesn't mean that you are seriously ill or certainly doesn't mean that you are a bad person or even possessed by evil forces if there are larger areas of congested life energy in your body. It just means that you're simply like everyone else. Perceive how you are at this moment, and you have created the most important prerequisite for your personal growth. You can only change what you consciously recognize. At the same time, it is a precondition for the meaningful interpretation of your subtle perception of other people that you can look at yourself to see how you are on this level.

In the spiritual realm, the path always leads from knowledge of the self to knowledge of the world. If you are seriously concerned about your state of health, then go to a healing practitioner in whom you trust and have an iris diagnosis done. On the one hand, this will help you realistically clarify the situation, and on the other hand you can check your own impressions when discussing the diagnosis. Equipped in this way, it will be easier for you to not be bothered by every block that you perceive within yourself.

In every session with the third exercise, you should dedicate special attention to one area of your body until you have a general survey of your current energetic state. Always take the front and back of the body into consideration in this and the following exercises. If you don't get done with an area in one session, continue with it the next time. Don't become insecure if you perceive a new dark spot at a later session or if old ones disappear. Take it as it is for the time being, and practice. I will explain this and other phenomenon in the next chapter.

Although this first impression of your momentary energy structure is still undifferentiated (the observation of various levels will follow later), it will still give you a good opportunity to come into contact with the practice of seeing the aura. For this reason, you should practice carefully and on a regular basis.

Exercise 4

Preparation: Same as for the last exercise.

Course of exercise: Do the HARA meditation for a number of breaths. Then look at yourself through your inner eyes using the heart look and select a certain region of your body that you want to work with more closely during this session. Now mentally formulate the desire to see areas that don't want to accept much energy covered in white. Pay attention to the change in your perception. Try not to interpret what you are seeing but immediately draw it on the blank form that you have ready next to you. End the exercise when the time has run out. Should you not be finished with looking at an area of the body, continue with it in the next session. Don't extend the sessions, even if they are very interesting!

At the end of every practice time, you should carry out the HARA meditation for a while. For this exercise as well, you should practice three minutes during the first week, five minutes a day in the second, and ten minutes in the third. Make a complete energy picture of your body in this way and transfer your perceptions from Exercise 3 and 4 onto the paper. This will be important later interpreting this black-and-white energram*.

Also note the date on which you have drawn this information on the page and that dates on which you have started with the Exercises 3 and 4. This documentation isn't meant to be for all eternity and it's very interesting to look at the old energrams after a time and compare them with the current one in order to recognize developments.

Exercise 5

Preparation: Same as for the last exercise.

Course of exercise: Do the HARA meditation for a moment and observe a larger area of your body using the heart look. Pay attention to light and dark places. Now mentally formulate the desire to see connections between blocks that are related to each other by way of black or white lines. Draw what you see on the form and don't get caught up in trying to interpret it. In order to keep things clear,

* By energram, I mean a sketch made during an aura-reading that depicts the flow and congestion of energy in the body. You will find an extensive form for this purpose in the appendix.

you can, for example, draw the dark connections as solid lines and the white connections as dashed lines. The length of the session should be as described under Exercise 4. This will make it easier for you later to work out precise interpretations and provides important help in dissolving blocks when you make energrams for other people. In addition, you have the possibility for yourself of learning much about your own personality structure. And we want to work with these experiences in the next chapter, which deals with the interpretation of an energram.

Summary

Learn the HARA meditation and check to what extent you can do it correctly with the test "The Iron Arm." After the first week of practice, start learning how to look with your heart. Exercise 1 and 2 form the absolutely necessary foundation for all further steps to seeing and interpreting auras. Only when you are secure in using both of these techniques should you start with the following exercises. Make a detailed energram of your body so that you have practical experience for understanding the theoretical explanations about the energy system of the human body in the next chapter. Do all the exercises carefully and on a regular basis, as described. In no case should you overdo it. Instead, learn to accept your own tempo. This will help your Inner Child develop more trust in you. It will work much more willingly with you if you accept its needs. You will ultimately learn more quickly and thoroughly in this way than with the "work morale" and "conquering your weaker self."

Chapter 4

Learning to Interpret the Aura

A Survey of the Human Energy System

Perceiving energetic processes and interpreting them in a meaningful way are two different pairs of shoes. If you don't know what information the black/white/gray pictures give you about the physical and emotional/mental condition of a person because you don't have an "encyclopedia" that tells you which observation has what concrete meaning, then reading auras won't do much for you and you must depend on presumptions with more or less of a foundation.

This is why this chapter deals with connections between body, mind, and soul and the significance of these connections for your health. Beginning with the muscle armor rings, which is a term based on bioenergetics, we will come to the seven main chakras and the most important secondary chakras through the energetic significance of the main organs and the meridians. In closing, we will explore the four basic fields of the aura.

However, in order to portray the human energy system in all its details and correlations, a library more extensive than the Encyclopedia Britannica would be necessary. There are thousands of fat volumes in the Tibetan monastery libraries on this topic. Although I would enjoy giving such a precise description, it would totally extend beyond the scope of this book and probably also exhaust your patience. So I have limited myself to a survey. In doing this, I find it important to discuss the interconnections between the various energetic levels and some principles of energy flow, which I explain in greater detail. I have made an effort to work out the most essential information and thereby give you a solid foundation for your own research work. In the bibliography, you will also find some good books on this topic if you want to take a closer look at the various aspects of the energy system. Unfortunately, I must hold back a few pieces of information here because it is only permissible to pass these on verbally. They aren't necessary for becoming familiar with reading auras either. When you have progressed so far in your development that you need this knowledge, you will definitely receive it in one way or another. This comment is just meant to explain some of the gaps in the description of the energy system.

If many of the statements in this chapter don't correspond with prevailing opinions, please try to understand. I would very much like for you to get practical use out of what I've written here, and this intention hasn't permitted me to be very considerate toward popular opinion. Please think seriously about what I've written and don't reject it immediately because you haven't heard things in quite this way before. This is how you can get the most use out of it. It's also a foregone conclusion that my system is just a map. It's a good and time-tested map, but just a map and not the landscape itself. And it's certainly not the only one that's right.

So now we can get started:

The Seven Armor Segments according to Wilhelm Reich

Among other things, the psychologist and natural scientist Wilhelm Reich focused on body mechanisms for holding back and storing undesired emotional energies. He discovered the muscle armor segments, which are included in treatment by practically all body-oriented psychotherapies today. These blocking mechanisms obstruct the natural flow of life, which shows itself in the body's process of "tension—charging—discharging—relaxation." In certain situations, it may be necessary to stop this flow. For example, when a child must obey its parents so that it isn't punished with deprivation of love because it has been "naughty." But if the stopping and freezing of the energy flow in a muscle group of the armor segment becomes a habit, a chronic tension behavior will result in time: Whenever a certain feeling wants to be expressed, a certain part of the body is tensed in order to inhibit or completely stop the flow of this energy. In the long run, this habit leads to decreased circulation and a reduced metabolism in the affected area of the body. Waste products and toxins are then deposited there since they can no longer be removed, and this is the basis for a susceptibility to many health disorders. In addition, chronic muscle armor not only has a direct effect within the afflicted region. All parts of the body are connected with

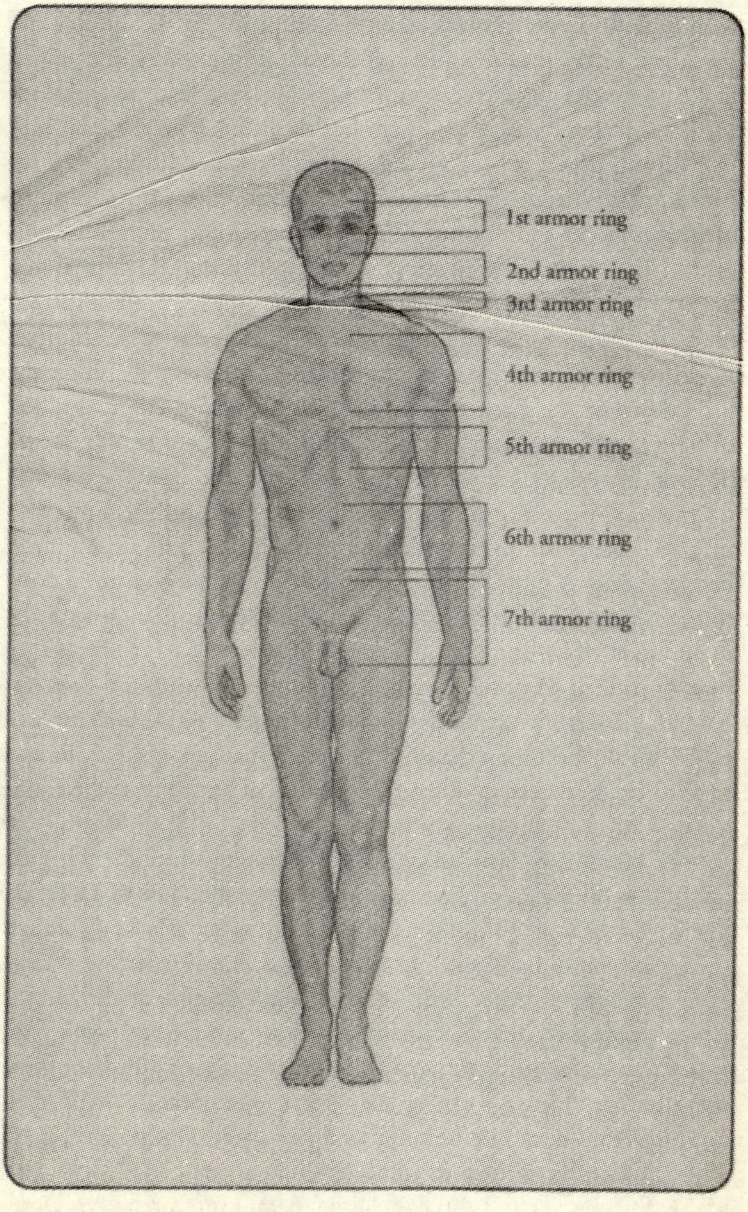

The Seven Armor Rings

each other through muscles, nerves, meridians, etc. If one area can no longer resonate and work with the others, then the others must make up for the defective function, which in turn leads to overloading and increased susceptibility to health disorders in the long run. The assumption is made in bioenergetics that in addition to the so-called primary block within which the emotion that cannot be lived out is frozen for some reason, a major block occurs in another area of the body. Energies are held onto here so that they don't reach the point of the primary block. Here secondary blocks result in turn to maintain the energetic equilibrium within the body. One example: A person constantly assumes a protective posture by bending the head down to the chest (primary block). If he now wants to look straight ahead or look up without changing the position of his head, he must tense certain muscle groups in the eye and back region (major block). As a result of this posture, the pelvis and legs must also assume other positions in order to maintain the equilibrium of the body (secondary blocks). In contrast to the naturally balanced position, this posture requires a great deal of muscle work in order to be maintained. The body must therefore employ a part of the energy that it produces in order to assume this tensed posture and does not have this energy available for other purposes. As a result, it will more quickly become exhausted in stress situations of all kinds and tend to become tired and produce feelings of reluctance when subject to a normal amount of strain.

The armor segments are arranged horizontally in rings. They do not necessarily include complete muscles, but often just that portion that lies on the ring. The streams of life energy, which may flow through the armor rings in a blocked or frozen form, flow vertically as vibrations through the body. The origin of these energies is the HARA region. From this point, they attempt to spread upward and downward.

In terms of reading the aura, it's important for you to confront this topic so that you can quickly survey the location, type, and extent of the blocked emotional energies when you do a reading. This can be of great help to you in evaluating energetic blocks with higher frequencies and also contribute to your interpretations closely approaching the reality of the situation. You will learn how to "filter out" the level of the armor segments in the next chapter. The prerequisite for this is becoming familiar with their significance and position. Look at the illustration on the opposite page.

The First Armor Ring
(Eyes-Ears)

Function: Sensory contact with the surrounding world through seeing and hearing. The information gets into the body without the necessity of taking in any substances. This means that these two senses are energy-oriented. Aggressions can't be overcome through these organs. An increase of attention can only be achieved by means of concentrating and thereby blocking other sensation qualities, as well as occupying as much of the mental capacity as possible with the preferred perception. At the level of the eyes, a reduction of attention is possible by closing them, concentrating on other sensations, or filtering out the undesired impressions. Physical defense mechanisms: impaired vision, becoming blind, as well as color-blindness (see chapter on meaning of colors). The attention of the ears can only be reduced by concentrating on other sensations or filtering out the undesired information. Physical defense mechanisms: limitation of ability to hear in sensitivity or frequency range; deafness.
Held emotions: fear of seeing or hearing a certain thing and being punished for it. Fear of not listening or seeing attentively enough and being punished for it.
Characteristic statements: I don't see and/or hear anything! I must see and/or hear it!

The Second Armor Ring
(Chin-Mouth-Throat-Upper-Neck-Nose)

Function: Sensory contact with the surrounding world through smell and taste. The information gets into the body through the absorption of substances. These two senses are therefore materially oriented. Physical defense mechanisms: among others, tensed jaw and mouth musculature (thin lips). Colds and sinusitis.
Held emotions: fear and anger at not being able to establish contact with the desired nourishment/relationship. Fear and anger at having to make contact with undesired nourishment/relationship.
Characteristic statements: I want physical contact with it! I don't want any physical contact with it!

The Third Armor Ring
(Neck Musculature-Tongue-Esophagus)

Function: Absorption of nourishment and experiencing its sensory quality through contact (tongue).

Held emotions: Fear and anger at not being able to incorporate desired nourishment/another being (in the figurative sense) and not being able to experience its sensory quality through contact (love deprivation).

Fear and anger at being forced (rape) to incorporate undesired nourishment/another being (in the figurative sense). Self-control in order to not have to show an aversion or desire.

Characteristic statements: I want to have that inside of me! I don't want to have that inside of me!

The Fourth Armor Ring
(Shoulder-Chest-Shoulder Blades)

Function: The body is provided with oxygen (material energy) and atmospheric Ki (subtle energy) through the respiration. It releases the transformed (used in relation to the body) material energy (carbon dioxide) and the transformed (used in relation to the body) atmospheric Ki. The lung is therefore an exchange organ that transfers important energies for the body in its metabolism and simultaneously expels energies that obstruct it. A posture like that of inhaling (pipe down!) is always assumed when undesired emotional energies are not (permitted) to be presented to the surrounding world and one's own consciousness. The body must then put these disruptive forces somewhere else. It uses the closest muscles for this purpose, which then become chronically tense (hardened) when this suppression takes place on a more frequent basis. This limits the overall ability to exchange energy.

Held emotions: emotional energies of all types are held onto here: anger, fear, aggression (wanting to make contact), sadness, suffering, longing, cheerfulness, hate, desire, wanting to embrace, reaching for something, etc.

Characteristic statement: I don't want myself and my surrounding world to perceive this part of me!

The Fifth Armor Ring
(Pit of the Stomach-Lower Ribs-Diaphragm-Stomach-Solar Plexus)

Function: The main respiratory muscle is found here with the diaphragm. In addition to breathing, the abdominal and pelvic organs are massaged through the free work of this muscle and emotional energies from this area are transmitted upward to the chest/shoulder region or downward into the abdominal/pelvic area. An unblocked diaphragm is an absolutely necessary precondition for the so-called "orgasm reflex," which means the free, lively, powerful vibrating and pulsating of the body in harmony with the stream of life energy.
Held emotions: desire; fear of desire; "yes"; devotion.
Characteristic statements: "No"; "I don't want to."

The Sixth Armor Ring
(Large Abdominal Muscle-Side Abdominal Muscle-Abdomen)

Function: Digestion takes place in the abdomen. The substances of nourishment necessary for the nutrition of the body are separated from those not beneficial to it and the former are transported into the inside of the body (strictly speaking, the intestines belong to the outside of the body!). The substances not suitable for the metabolism are transported out of the body (detoxification).
Held emotions: desire for detoxification; fulfillment; self-assurance.
Characteristic statements: I am not happy/fulfilled/satisfied!

The Seventh Armor Ring
(Entire Pelvic Area-Buttocks-Genital Organs)

Function: Seat of the genital and excretory system. On the one hand, new life can be conceived in this area of the body, vibrations of desire, life, and power can be produced, and satisfaction experienced; on the other hand, substances and energies that aren't tolerable for the body can be released.
Held emotions: liveliness, love of life, joy, oneness with the universe through resonance in the universal stream of life, eroticism and sexuality, fear and anger in relation to these feelings.
Characteristic statement: "I don't want to flow along in the stream of liveliness. I need goals, rules, and order, and someone to tell me what's good for me!"

Note: Because of the essential importance of the pelvic area for a person's liveliness and health, I would like to give some further explanations on the process that take place here. A pelvis that isn't blocked is a RECEIVER for energies from the surrounding world, which a human being requires for maintaining his or her physical and mental/emotional vital functions on all levels. These energies are produced by other living beings in their own special quality and, because they can't use these energies themselves, released so that other beings, for whom these forces are vital for life, can absorb and use them. These in turn can release the energies in their transformed state once again in order to supply them to other life forms. The pelvic region thereby serves simultaneously as a TRANSMITTER for such transformed energies. A graphic example of this process is the utilization of carbon dioxide by plants, which require the carbon that it contains for their own metabolism and release oxygen back into the environment. Animals and human beings need this oxygen for their metabolism, using carbon to change it into carbon dioxide, and give this combination back to the surrounding world again so that it is available to the plants for their vital processes. Panta rhei—everything flows! If the pelvis tends to be blocked, these functions that are necessary for life will then be obstructed. A reduced sense of liveliness, feelings of unhappiness, and a state of lacking fulfillment occur. In the exchange, in the flow of energies lies cheerfulness, happiness, and life. Holding on is the basis of death.

The Correlation Between the Armor Rings

As already mentioned above, many other blocks are created in the various regions of the body as a result of the original blocks. Every human is a unique being, which is why there are no generally valid rules for the structure of these blocks. On the other hand, experience has shown that certain blocked rings frequently correspond with others.

So that you have an insight into the cross-linking possibilities, I would like to provide a brief description of the most important connections.

Because of their function in making sensory contact with the surrounding world, the first and second armor rings are closely linked.

If one of these blocks is relaxed, the congestion is frequently increased in the other.

Both of the first two armor rings are linked with the fifth armor segment (diaphragm area). Example: A person perceives a situation that he has learned to interpret as threatening (producing fear). He immediately senses a queasy feeling in his stomach area (solar plexus-diaphragm).

The second armor segment is connected with the seventh armor ring (pelvic region). Example: The intimate contact during a French kiss produces sexual arousal. Aversion against kissing often shows a far-reaching aversion against genital contact. There is also the vicarious function: eating instead of sexual satisfaction. The excretory function is also reflected in both segments: If a substance not beneficial for the body still manages to get inside of the body, it will be eliminated either through vomiting or diarrhea.

The third armor ring (neck) with its function of self-control ("choking" off feelings/needs) has a close relationship with the fourth, fifth, and seventh armor rings. These blocks mutually support each other in the defense/storage of undesired lively energy vibrations (also compare the description of the meaning of the neck and pelvic posture for the ability of the body to resonate in Chapter 2).

A sadistic/masochistic attitude toward life also has its seat in the functional unity of these blocks. I define this attitude not as a certain form of sexual lifestyle but rather as the will, which has grown out of the fear of punishment, to regulate one's own way of living (masochism) or other people's way of living (sadism) according to certain laws and givens instead of leaving this up to the respective person's own living desires and needs. As long as someone tries to follow a certain diet, philosophy of life, plan for spiritual growth, physical exercises, etc. without being concerned about whether or not these activities are enjoyable, he or she more or less lives with a masochistic/sadistic basic attitude toward life. A typical symptom for this in esoteric circles is the orientation toward so-called higher goals and service to the people around us. Tending to give up one's own personal needs and own path in life in favor of fulfilling a fictitious task for the good of humanity (who asked humanity if it even wants this?) or caring for others (why shouldn't another people be permitted to have experiences in their own way and why should they have to be missionized?) ultimately contributes to general unhappiness. No one finds personal fulfillment by doing something for others that they should be doing for themselves instead. When the flow of a person's life energy is congested for the purpose of making other people feel better or rescuing them, such relationships always leave behind the stale taste of dependence. What are the rescuers of humanity doing when they should be saving themselves?

The fourth armor ring is linked with the third and fifth. It conveys the energy surpluses that one segment cannot hold to the other segment and serves thereby as an intermediate storage (pulling up the shoulders when fears arise), as well as the place of "final storage" (chronically tensed shoulders).

The fifth armor ring (diaphragm) radiates to all the other blocked rings because of its essential function of respiration. This is particularly pronounced in the relationship to the pelvic segment. In both block structures, a fundamental coupling of the energy exchange with the surrounding world exists. Both have close contact with the pulsating life stream of the universe.

The sixth armor ring has a function similar to the fourth in relation to both the armor segments five and six located in its immediate vicinity. Holding back emotions of all types can be expressed here through constipation, for example. Diarrhea and inflammation of the intestines can help get rid of energies that shouldn't be lived out or express them in a way that appears to be less dangerous to the conscious mind. If a person can't get rid of the bothersome life impulses in this way either, then he will possibly put himself in the hands of a specialist who takes the part overloaded with undesired energy out of the body (for example: removal of the appendix, the prostate gland, and the ovaries).

Like the diaphragm segment, the seventh armor ring is connected with all others. However, this contact is even more profound and extensive. Although it is quite possible to dissolve the diaphragm block while there are still other blocks, a fundamental harmonization of the pelvic area is impossible without the complete dissolving of all(!) other blocks. If the continuous flow of the life stream is still obstructed somewhere in the body, there is a back-up and the transmitter/receiver function of the pelvis is more or less disrupted. This fact also results in an energetic connection with the seventh chakra, the crown chakra, the energy center that can also only be completely developed when a person has learned to completely love on the level of the other chakras. More about this later.

The Level of the Organs

The level of the armor segments is very close to the material body in the energetic sense. The following organ level in my system is somewhat more subtle. Please don't confuse this level with the material organ level, which is connected with the energetic level but superordinate to it. For this reason, I don't want to go into extensive detail about the medical anatomy and function of the organs. If you are interested in this aspect, please look at the bibliography in the appendix. I have listed a number of good books on the subject there.

The energetic function of the organs has been part of the Asian tradition for a long time. Knowledge of this energetic function is used in such methods as acupuncture therapy and Tao Yoga. I have worked with the Chinese system for many years, and have been able to determine time and again that it's very good at doing justice to the practice. In addition, it has the advantage of an extensive theoretical superstructure (I Ching, Taoist alchemy, astrology, etc.) and many practical techniques (inner martial arts, Tao Yoga, Qi Gong, acupuncture, etc.) that are built upon it. This is why I pass it on here, along with some small changes resulting from my personal experience.

The meaning of the energetic quality of the organs can be easily derived from the Chinese theory of five elements. This also makes a good starting point for interpreting the condition of the chakra system with the I Ching, an ancient Chinese oracle that I will describe in Chapter 6.

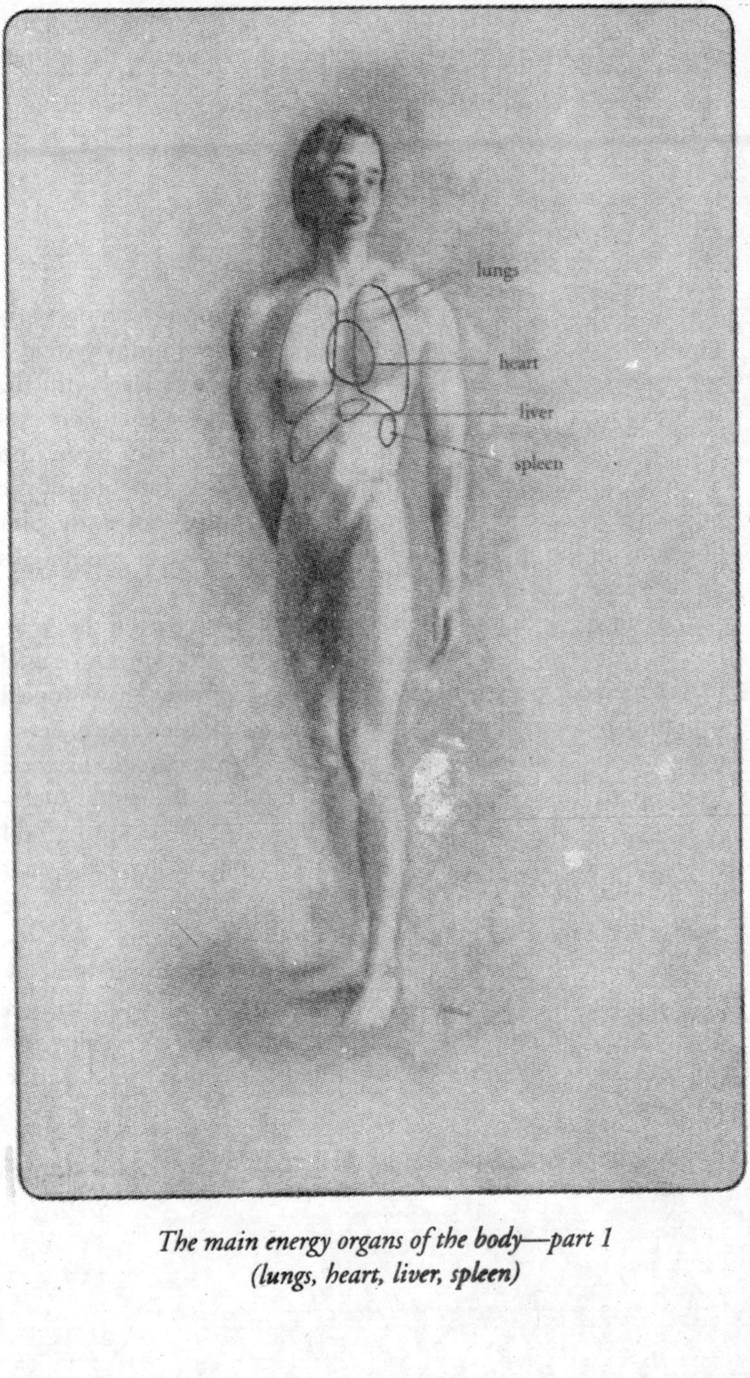

The main energy organs of the body—part 1
(lungs, heart, liver, spleen)

The Function of the Five Main Energetic Organs

Heart

Element: Fire

Function: The heart is the connection to the vibrations of universal life energy. As long as this connection is fundamentally permitted, a human being is in a state of basic trust in the depths of his or her personality. In the Christian tradition, this "trust in God" is expressed by the words of the Psalm "The Lord is my shepherd, I shall not want...," for example. If the conviction that I will get what I need is anchored within me, then I won't have a desire for a good "bargain," quick sex, quick money, and a quick acquisition of power. This attitude is called "morality" by Chinese medicine. The certainty that everything will come to me at the time that I truly need it makes hoarding and senseless sensory pleasures (because they are not appropriate for me at the moment) undesirable. A life lived from the heart makes laws and morality superfluous. Regulation from the outside can only imperfectly replace self-regulation. A blocked heart is a reason for a more or less deep insecurity, a mistrust of the world and ultimately of oneself. People who need "proof" of another person's love in order to feel secure in a relationship or live according to the saying "trust is good, control is better!" may have an energetic block in the heart, among other things.

On the organic level, the heart is a pump that keeps the blood, a human being's sap of life, in movement. It ensures proper distribution of the nutrients, essential energies, information bearers, and naturally oxygen, and that the defensive cells as the police of the body remove the toxins and waste products created in the metabolic processes. If the physical vibration that is also shown in the rhythmically alternating readiness to expand and constrict the blood vessels (yin and yang!) harmonizes the heart rhythm on the whole, then the supply and disposal works well. If the physical rhythm deviates greatly from the universal rhythm because of arbitrary obstruction or control of the lifestyle, the heart must increasingly strain itself and will somehow lose the proper rhythm or wane in its strength after a certain amount of time. However, such organic effects generally require many years before they have worked their way through the body's energetic buffer system. Much strength and time is necessary to detach oneself from the vibration of love.

When a person has recognized that he lives against his own health in this respect, he can get back into better contact with the creative force in a relatively easy and expedient way: by replacing concentration and assertion of will with the direction of attention in order to permit more consciousness and the use of the intellect in order to enable living out the natural needs of the body-mind-soul in an optimal way. Therapy for the heart involves harmonizing the energies of cruelty (also or particularly toward oneself), hastiness (rushing past a fulfilled life because of fear), and impatience (the fear of not accomplishing enough on time and being punished for it). These energies should in no case be suppressed. Instead, their roots must be understood through a far-reaching process of becoming conscious and the satisfaction of existing needs in a holistically meaningful manner.

Thank your body that it tries to fulfill its (and therefore also your) needs in the respectively best possible way, as long as you couldn't or didn't want to help with the conscious part of your self. By the way, excessive use of strong stimulants of all types is also based on a block in the heart region. The motto of our time "faster, higher, further!" clearly shows a tendency in our society toward a congestion in the heart meridian. So don't be surprised if you frequently determine held energy in this area.

Within this context, it's also interesting to compare the virtually obsessed way in which many Western artists work with the contemplative/meditative manner of the creative process in the Asian tradition of art (for example, Zen painting and ikebana). Free, spontaneous laughing (not laughing at someone or gloating!) can be very effective in helping to loosen the energetic blocks in the heart. The heart has an energetic connection to the tongue and to a human being's acoustic expressions, which can be used for therapeutic and diagnostic purposes.

Kidneys

Element: Water

Function: The kidneys regulate the energy in relationships. And this includes not only relationships directed toward the outside but also those of a human being with himself like the body consciousness, the consciousness of one's own roots (tradition, family, profession,

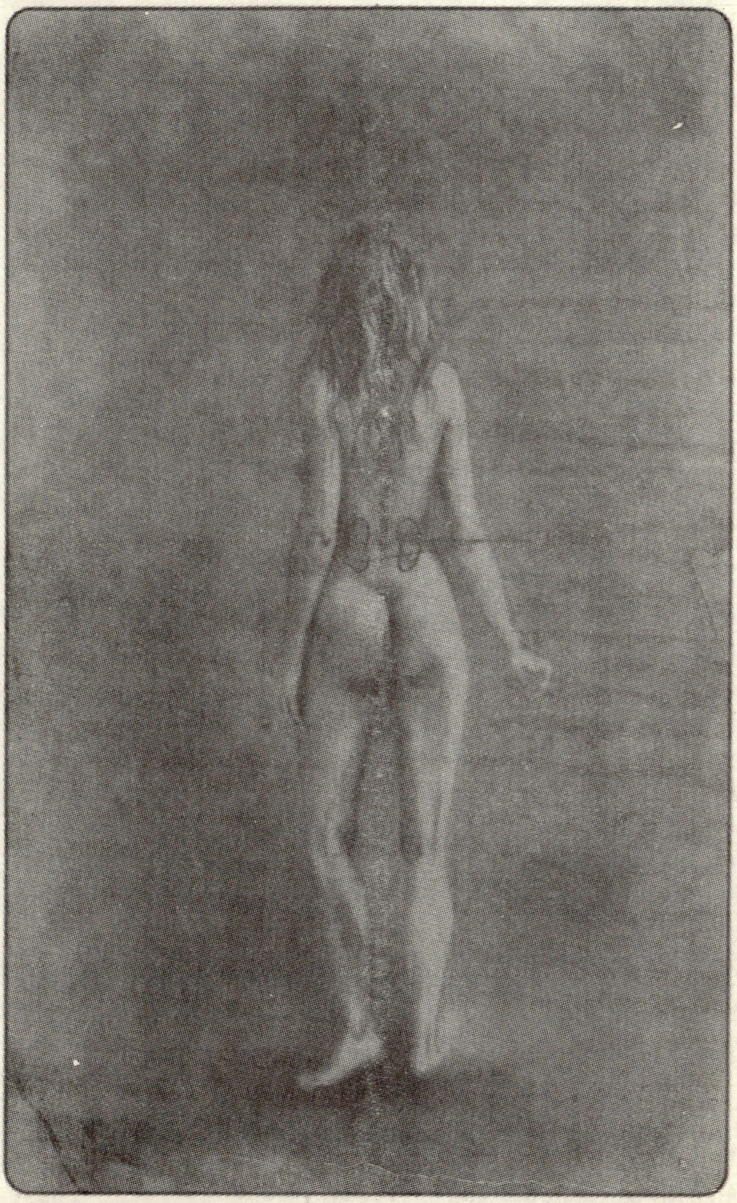

The main energy organs of the body—part 2 (kidneys)

nationality or race, etc.). Chinese medicine attributes to the **kidneys** the quality of being a bearer of hereditary energies, meaning the power potential that a person has from his or her ancestry (which includes not only the physical ancestors but the spiritual as well) at the time of birth. This power potential is inexhaustible if a person makes the efforts to live out these talents, as these energies can also be called, in the holistic context. It tends to become exhausted or a person detaches himself from this potential, which basically cannot be used up, when he shapes his life in such a way that it becomes increasingly impossible to develop his talents through the structures that he has created for himself. If someone constantly lives against the task in life that he chose before this incarnation, he drains his rather limited personal energies and must exert himself greatly to accomplish what he wants. Fast careers with a sudden, drastic collapse are created, among other things, from a block of the kidneys in connection with a heart block. In this situation, the kidney talents are practically exploited without being attuned to the rhythm of the universe in their tempo of realization by the stabilizing energy of the heart. After a certain time, the energetic mechanism responsible for realizing hereditary energies fails because it is overloaded.

An excessive sex life also belongs to this disturbance region. I don't mean frequent and satisfying sexual encounters on a regular basis but a life that is essentially determined by sex without profound satisfaction and the feeling of harmony and fulfillment during and after the contact.

In a man, the storage of the personal sexual energy is ascribed to the left kidney, meaning the powers that provide a newborn with its hereditary energy. In a woman, this energy is stored in the right kidney. Through fulfilled sexual relationships and spiritual development within one's own tradition (which every individual must find for himself), this power is strengthened. Through this association, the connection of the left kidney with the prostate gland and testicles in the man and the right kidneys with the ovaries and uterus in a woman becomes easier to understand. There is also a relationship to body consciousness and to one's own Inner Child.

The right kidney in the man and the left kidney in the woman have a connection to external relationship partners and accordingly tends to be strengthened through harmonious relationships and weakened through inharmonious relationships. In addition, these organs regulate the intensity of contacts in relationship to their significance for one's own path in life. When friendships end without the participants being able to really explain why, this is a result of the kidneys' guidance. The same applies to love at first sight, the heart connection between teacher and student that both become aware of even after a brief acquaintance, and also the spontaneous hiring of employees or the intuitive desire to work at a certain enterprise or in a specific project.

The tasks of the two kidneys naturally aren't separated as strictly as I have described them here. The transitions are more or less flowing, but with the orientation emphasis mentioned above. It is important for you to feel your way into this area, which isn't all that simple. To do this, compare the kidney disorders in your own biography and the lives of others with the model depicted above. Don't be satisfied with superficial reasons but research until you have found truly satisfying answers. At the same time, be sure to respect the private lives and vulnerabilities of others and don't pounce on them with your interpretations.

On the organic level, the kidneys have the task of filtering out substances not beneficial for the body and eliminating them through the urinary passages (break off relationships that don't correspond to your own needs!). In addition, they play an important role in the regulation of the blood pressure and the water and salt metabolism in the body, the buffering of energies of the liver (blood pressure), which is responsible for delivering creative power for the realization of talents. These are then "modulated" accordingly by the kidneys and released at the request of the heart (letting water flow) or held back (salt retains water).

In energetic therapy, it is necessary to harmonize the fear that stops a person from entering into the relationships that correspond to him and build him up, and let himself find fulfillment within them. This fear often results from a life program that has been learned (you must work at this profession, have such and such a partner, have this kind of person as a friend, etc.), which is anchored under threat of punishment in one way or another deep within the character of a human being. To the same extent, there is frequently also the fear of living relationships that are "right" for the respective person in a certain way because this type of lifestyle is put under a taboo for some reason.

A shock can also block the kidneys. If it is intense enough, it can even cause organic failure, which can quickly lead to death. I define this type of shock as a reaction to a sudden, actual or presumed threat to physical or emotional/mental intactness in a relationships that is felt to be essentially secure. This kidney trauma often occurs "out of the blue" after serious accidents in an acute or more chronic form, such as the realization that the companion in life has had or is having sexual contact with a third person.

One possibility for healing the kidneys is contact with wisdom. An oracle like the I Ching, the Tarot, or runes, as well as a good psychotherapist or a truly spiritual teacher, can help the person with the health disorder perceive the meaning of his or her life, lovingly accept it, and translate it into reality for the benefit of the entire Creation. In this way, difficult relationships (even with oneself!) can become a life-shaping creative process that virtually cause a person to blossom. In healing the kidneys, it's important to be sure that no overly intellectual pseudo-development through reading books or lonesome meditation and the like takes place. Since the kidneys represent the relationship organ of a human being, their blocked energies can also be freed only through relationships. So long-term work on a regular basis with a psychotherapist/spiritual teacher cannot be replaced, but only complemented, by individual work. The kidneys have an energetic connection to the abdomen, the ears, and the sense of hearing, which can be made use of in a therapeutic and diagnostic sense.

Liver

Element: Wood

Function: The liver is the energy organ of the body. It makes available all types of aggressive powers and gives the process of personal realization the pressure it needs. The manipulation of reality for the creation of a new, tolerable overall situation is its task. Without this force, the ideas get stuck in the planning stage and aren't used to structure the Creation. Aggression is often confused with destructive violence today and made taboo for this reason. But the fact is that aggressive energy only becomes destructive and inharmonious when a person doesn't consciously accept his dynamic power and employ it sensibly within the holistic context. Since aggression doesn't allow itself to be turned off or transformed, the only possibilities are for it to be lived out in a meaningful way or congested in the muscle armor or other buffers in the body until their capacity is overloaded or the control mechanism that normally functions is switched off (intense stress, fear, greed, herd instinct—for example, at demonstrations or sport events). Only in these two latter cases does this force of the personality, which is constructive in its basic nature, become harmful. Then its violence becomes just like a dam that is filled to the brim breaks and sweeps away everything blocking its flow. People with chronically congested vital energy frequently like to look for scapegoats who "are to blame for (...)" so that they have someone on whom they can "justifiably" work out their aggressions. People who seem peaceful enough to the outside world can turn into rapacious beasts when they've found the "right one." Examples of this that come to mind are the many bloody confrontations in the name of peace, religious beliefs, or ideologies.

In organic terms, the liver has the function of an extensive chemistry lab. It converts substances that are unnecessary at the moment into the best possible required substances. It detoxifies substances dangerous to the metabolism by chemically transforming them, serves as an intermediate storage place for quickly utilizable energy, produces digestive juices to process the food in a way that the body can put them to good use, and directs toxins and waste materials out of the body through the gallbladder.

In energetic terms, the liver also supplies the aggressive components of sexuality. Sexuality's other components, those of unification, are contributed by the kidneys. Sexuality cannot be separated from this dynamic force, which isn't even necessary to do when it's accepted. Mind you—I'm not talking about sadomasochistic relationships or machismo here! The aggressive components of sexual energy are absolutely necessary for the manipulation of substances and primal energies if a new living being is to be created. For this procedure to take place in a meaningful way, the aggressive energy of the liver is provided with the proper modulations by the kidneys in a time-related process determined by the heart. When the liver energy is lived out in a harmonious way between sexual partners, it makes sure that their sexual desires are aroused. Just like the kidneys with their wish for unity make sure that we meet the right partner, the liver produces a strong emotional attraction (which, by the way, is the original meaning of the word "aggression"!) that can lead to a longer-term partnership and sexual contacts between the two people.

When the liver energy isn't lived out in a meaningful way, this is expressed in such problems as blood pressure that is too high or too low, congestion of blood in the head, poor circulation within the individual parts of the body that have the task of satisfying certain needs that aren't permitted, or severe tenseness (muscle armor rings!). If you want to harmonize the liver energy, first create possibilities for yourself of living out this strong force, without harming others, in order to reduce the surplus collected over a long period of time. This is important in order to free yourself from the vicious circles of blame. No one other than yourself is responsible for your rage. Accept this responsibility and you will start off on a completely new, productive, fulfilled, and self-determined life. An experienced body therapist (bioenergetics, Reichian body work, Scan, Core energetics, for example) can be very helpful in this process.

Once you have gradually broken down your "mountain of rage," you can start learning to apply your aggressive energies in a meaningful way when they arise. This will help you avoid a new syndrome of congested energy. Oracle work, psychotherapy, working with a spiritual teacher, or even martial arts training (such as Aikido, Tai Chi Chuan, Hsing I) with an experienced, responsible teacher can help you here. Healing the liver is a matter of harmonizing the feeling of rage. Rage grows from the fear of not being able to achieve self-realization.

A lifestyle that corresponds to an individual tends to reduce the rage and directs this force within him into other, more constructive qualities of aggression. Through mental and practical occupation with the attribute of kindness, the liver energy can be harmonized. I understand "kindness" within this context to be the quality that attempts to let all participants in a situation get something useful for themselves in the holistic sense. You can also compare this with my comments in *Reiki—Way of the Heart*, (Lotus Light/Shangri-La), about the cosmic laws of fair energy exchange. As an aside, there is a strong energetic connection between the liver and the feet (making progress!). This interrelation can be put to therapeutic and diagnostic use.

Lungs

Element: Metal

Function: The lungs and the heart represent two receivers that complement each other for the body-mind-soul of a human being. As you remember, the heart is the connection to the vibration of unity in the universe, to the source of all life. The energy vibration that it receives is basically always the same. This is non-polar and imparts the information about the eternal rhythm of becoming on the one level of being and passing away on the other level of being, which is determined by the previous one and vice versa. If a person orients himself toward this pulsation of the universe, the energies and substances of the surrounding world that he has imprinted (for example, carbon dioxide, material possessions, ideas and their realization), which are needed at the moment in order to fulfill his tasks in the universal context of the infinitely flowing process of Creation, will be available to him on all levels of his personality. The materialization of this productive exchange of energy is the task of the lungs. If they function in the rhythm set by the heart, the body's processes of energy intake and output will be optimally coordinated with each other and attuned with the requirements of the surrounding world. This can also be compared with the relaxing effect of auto-suggestion in autogenous training: "it's breathing me." I trustingly leave the control of my lung activity up to my heart and therefore don't need to strain (tense) myself in order to maintain the necessary exchange process.

The organic correlations of the lung activity with the circulation (through the control of the kidneys in part) also leads to interesting information. The lung is therefore a communication organ. If its function is disrupted, the respective individual will have difficulties with the process of exchange. These imbalances are usually expressed in a tendency toward an "overly mental" lifestyle: specific diets, physical exercises, and/or breathing exercises are carried out without any consideration of the emotional needs or even attempting to feel to the desires of the body. This act of self-violation is often justified by theories about health and the realization of ideological systems that are meant to serve a "higher goal." The root of this disorder can be found in a childhood characterized by disciplinary measures and/or the fear of resonating and flowing along in the stream of life (diaphragm and pelvic armor!). Flowing along would mean giving up safe positions. This is unconsciously linked with a free fall into nothing, meaning death. It's understandable that a fear reaching down to the roots of an incarnation isn't so easy to give up.

Even the decision to strive to find out the reasons for such symptoms is usually preceded by an enormous expenditure of energy, usually because of the intensive pressure of suffering. If you determine that someone has such an energetic disorder of the lung function, treat your client like a raw egg! Respect the fear of death that he has lurking in his unconscious mind and don't pounce on him with deep analysis and advice. When there is a block of the lungs, only a slow, cautious approach to these problems is possible. If you do not have the appropriate qualifications, your counseling should only prepare the way and lead up to a therapy with a sensitive professional (psychotherapist) who is familiar with this type of disorder.

The feelings of sadness, worry, and depression (often connected with weakness, sleep disorders, aversion against sexuality, and other consequences of a detachment from the universal exchange processes) are the result of an Inner Child (body consciousness) that is strongly obstructed in its desires, that isn't permitted to play, and is always kept "under house arrest." In theory, all methods that let the consciousness enter into contact with the desires of the body or strengthen the self-regulating abilities of the organism are suitable in order to resolve lung blocks. Examples of these methods are Reiki, particularly the mental-healing techniques of the Second Degree, intuitive breathing work, Tai Chi Chuan, Aikido, Vipassana meditation, Zen meditation, Three-Ray meditation, and fantasy journeys into the inside of the body, supplemented by conversations with the organs.

All forms of intensely confrontational therapy and meditation methods should be avoided, particularly during the first phase, since an attitude of refusal may be provoked within the respective person. Who would want to be pushed out of the tenth floor? Contemplation and a conscious life of justice (letting everyone and everything have what they deserve!) can also help in dissolving blocks in the lungs. The lungs are energetically connected with the ears, the nose, and the skin (contact with the outer world!). These relationships can be put to therapeutic and diagnostic use.

Spleen

Element: Earth

Function: The spleen is the architect of the organism. According to the directions given by the kidneys, heart, and lungs, it takes care of converting the liver energy into a form beneficial for these organs. It represents a significant part of grounding with subtle energies of the body. A person with a blocked spleen has more or less severe difficulties in living in accordance with his theoretical knowledge and his strongly felt desire for life. "I know what I should do, but I don't know how I should it!" is a typical remark for these symptoms. He doesn't know what to make of himself and the world. Armchair planners and the ivory-tower scientists are metaphors for people with spleen blocks. Brooding, doubting, and deliberating (racking their brains) are typical occupations for them. Since they never get to the point of having intense, practical experiences with the topic of their pondering, their discussions for pro and con never stop. The ideology of the scholars who seriously discussed how many angels could fit on the tip of a needle also fits into this realm.

But energy congestion in the spleen also has physical consequences. Since it doesn't bring the energies and instructions of the other organs together in a harmonious manner and let them become concrete, the detoxification system of the body and the defense against germs and outside energies tends to be disturbed. The weakness of the immune system is reflected by the weakness of the aura. Such an individual doesn't have any personal magnetism—no charisma. A person with a completely functional spleen that materializes the energies and instructions of the other, also completely functional organs, is in a state of holiness. Through the actions that he takes—or doesn't take—he brings God, the universal creative will, or whatever you want to call it, to the earth. He is strong, kind, just, loving, wise, and moral (in the Chinese sense!). All beings thrive through him. But once achieved, the state of enlightenment doesn't unconditionally last forever. It also isn't particularly unusual. If all of us weren't holy or enlightened from time to time, nothing would work anymore in the world. "God has only our hands" according to the Sufi tradition. If you want to see it this way, the spiritual hand of God is the spleen when it functions as it should. This is why all processes of renewal belong to the spleen's tasks on the organic level. Cancer can therefore fundamentally be attributed to a block of this organ, but always also in connection with severe disorders in other main functional organs of the body. A link between a disrupted functioning of the spleen and a cancer-promoting mucous obstruction in the body was already known to Paracelsus and has been confirmed by modern medicine. AIDS is also strongly related to the spleen. Diabetes, in which sugar (a metaphor for the sweetness of life) can't be utilized by the body and therefore must be eliminated through the urine, also has its cause in a certain type of spleen block.

Enlightenment is, as already mentioned, not necessarily a continual state. It always stubbornly eludes its realization when I absolutely want to have it since asserting my will impedes the assertion of the divine will. No one can serve two masters at the same time. A possibility for releasing a spleen block is free artistic work, using with the clay box according to Dürckheim, or intuitive painting. Any type of guided creative work is basically suitable for an energetic healing of the spleen. In the beginning phase, a very sensitive instruction of the client, which has neither too many nor too few parameters, is necessary. With the progress of the healing process, the work can increasingly turn into working together; an ideal result of such therapy is independent, harmonious creativity.

The cause of a chronic spleen block may be feelings that one's own abilities are inadequate in comparison with a significant adult. There is an important energetic connection between the spleen and the lips, tongue muscles, teeth, and the hands. This can be put to therapeutic and diagnostic use. Take a moment to think about the possible correlations between smoking, kissing, and, for example, the "dry lips" that apparently lack the water element (where else does this belong?). If the spleen is removed by way of an operation, the liver will take over its energetic and organic tasks after a shorter or longer transitional phase. However, the liver doesn't take them over completely. A deficit will remain. If other main organs are strengthened, the deficit can be reduced even more.

The Fourteen Main Meridians

Following the main organs and their energetic function for the human being, we now go further in the subtle area to the fourteen main meridians. The connections of the five main organs with each other and with the performing organs are created, as well as the harmonization of their yin and yang portions in two special meridians. These are the energy-conducting pathways of the body. Moreover, the meridians are energy storage places and can assume functions similar on the subtle-energetic levels to those of the muscle armor rings described above. However, the meridians store not only undesired energy—they also serve the rhythmic organization of the body processes by collecting specific energies for a period of time and then more intensely releasing the collected surplus over a certain time span. This creates, for example, the phenomenon of the organ clock, which is explained in the theory of acupuncture. This means that certain organs have an intensified function that is followed by a period of weakened functioning at regularly recurrent time periods.

In the following section, I have given a brief summary of the tasks of the individual meridians, without going into greater detail about them. These details aren't absolutely necessary for the practice of reading auras, unless you work therapeutically in this area—and if this is the case, you will already know about them. If you would like to have additional special information about the meridians, read the books listed under this topic in the bibliography.

However, for the practice of reading auras it can be very useful if you know the course of the meridians. The three illustrations on the preceding pages can help you in getting oriented on the meridian level. You don't need to learn them by heart. Since you (hopefully) prepare an energram of every aura-reading, as discussed in Chapter 3, you can use the meridian sketches afterward to help determine exactly which meridians you have seen. It's not very practical to classify specific meridians in an improvised manner when doing a reading, except if you have much practical experience in this area and have thoroughly worked your way into it.

The Liver Meridian

Collecting and releasing the dynamic, creative, "hard-working" energies is the task of the liver meridian, the power plant of the body. In

the case of functional disorders, weakness, a lack of physical and/or mental resistance to stress, or—precisely the opposite situation—exaggerated, confused activity may occur. An enthusiasm for work, resolution, the ability to digest, and aggressions have their origin here.
Works together with: Gallbladder meridian.
Correction through: Lung meridian.
Element: Wood (interestingly enough, the Chinese medical philosophy sees aggressive energy in relation to healthy growth and liveliness. The frequently encountered opinion in the West that aggression is harmful and not in the sense of the universal order generally isn't found in this form in this teaching. The Chinese views are much more comprehensive.)
Associated feelings: Content/worried.
Qualities: Vitality, emotion, dynamism, and/or their opposite counterparts.

The Heart Meridian

The development of individuality within the scope of the cosmic order through collecting and releasing special energies in relation to the personality, as they stand in the plan for life that has been established before birth is the task of the heart meridian. This includes the rhythmic flow of the vital energies; the regulation of phases such as recuperation, work, sleep, and being awake; the connection of the body-mind-soul on the material level with the source of all life on the superordinate level. The main effect is on the level of the feelings, the intellect, and the psyche.
Works together with: Small intestine meridian.
Controlled by: Kidney meridian.
Element: Fire (Fire is characterized by heat, a strong ability to react to environmental stimuli such as a draft of air, dynamism, and the direct conditionality in terms of a material fuel. If there is no more material, the fire goes out. This little sketch can help you understand why we are incarnated here on the earth: Without to connection to the material world (fuel) and the unification of opposites (process of burning), no enlightenment, no blossoming of the ability to love (flame) can be achieved. We are not here to atone for some debt but because there would be no progress in the development of the entire universe and all the other levels, often called the higher subtle levels, without this level.)

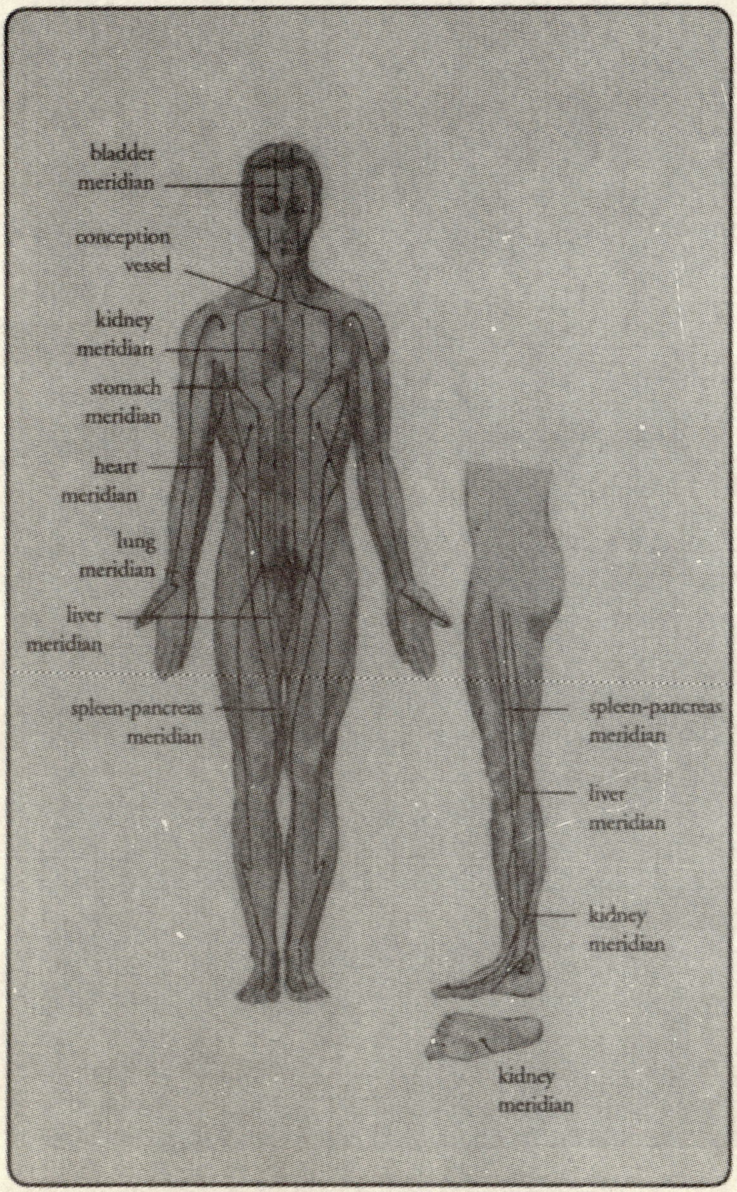

The main meridians of the body—illustration part 1

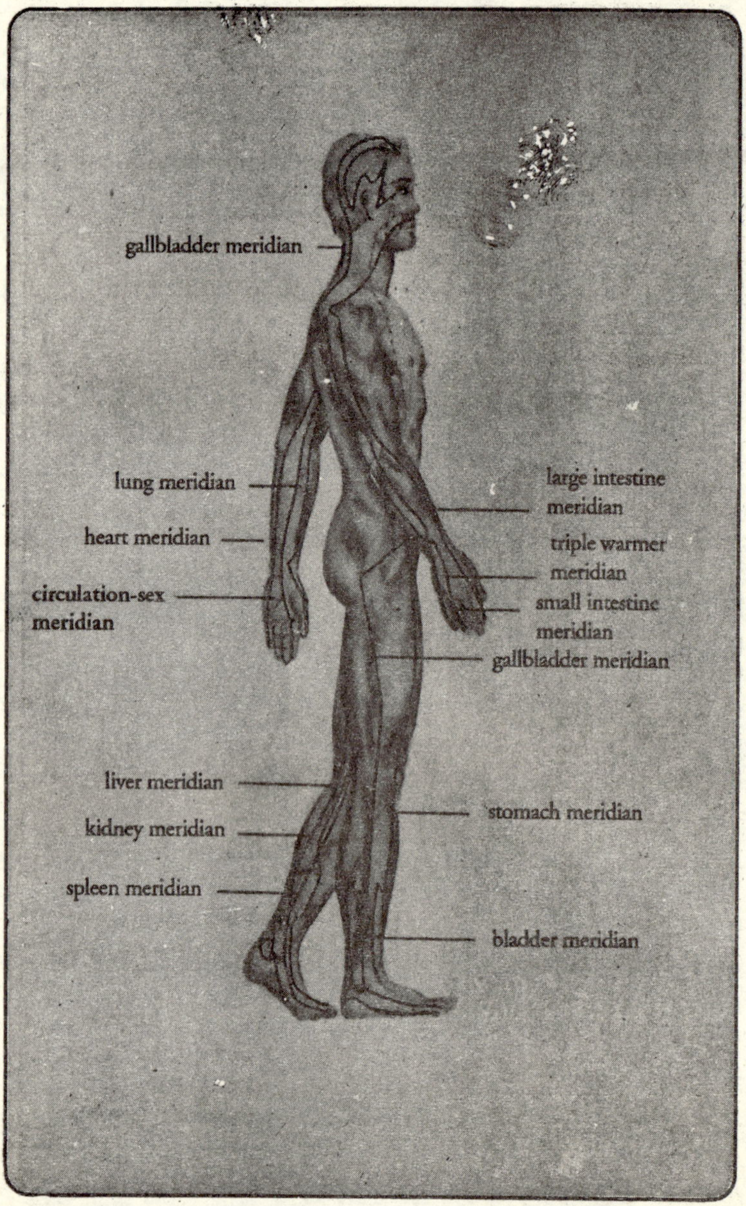

The main meridians of the body—illustration part 2

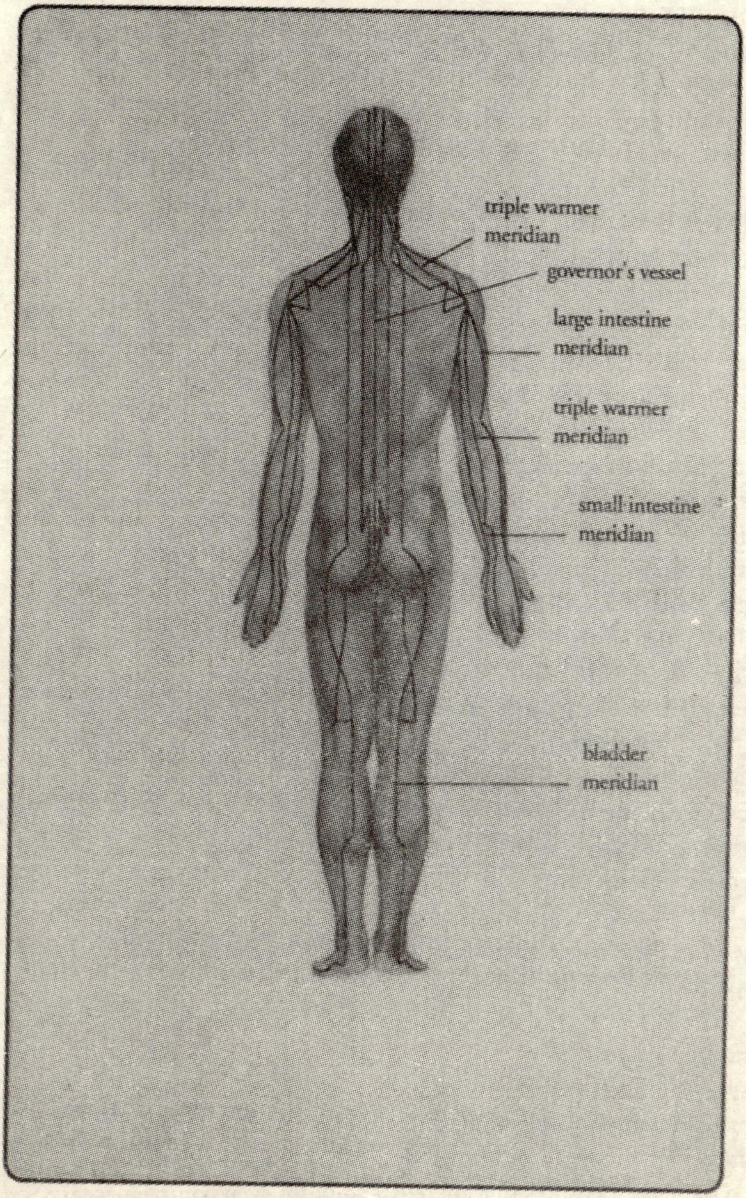

The main meridians of the body—illustration part 3

Assigned feelings: Secure/insecure.
Qualities: Joy, desire, love, unity, and/or their opposite counterparts.

The Spleen-Pancreas Meridian

This functional cycle makes sure that every region of the body-mind-soul receives the energies and substances that it needs in order to fulfill its tasks. This also means that all influences from the outside somehow come into contact with this meridian and are classified by it. The pattern according to which this process takes place is learned for the most part. This is why human beings are so flexible and can adapt themselves to a great variety of environmental conditions, above all when they are young and the spleen-pancreas meridian hasn't yet been as strongly encumbered by "programs." To this extent, it is also the seat of the acquired constitution in contrast to the kidney meridian, which is involved with the physically and emotionally inherited traits, among other things. If this meridian functions well, a person can easily and quickly adapt to new situations and deal with them well. If it is disturbed, the adaptability and ability to react is reduced in accordance with the disorder. This functional cycle with its structuring work also ensures that we remain true to ourselves at the center of our personality under changing external conditions. In this respect, an overall stabilizing power also originates here. Neuroses of all types are generally related to this functional cycle.
Works together with: Stomach meridian.
Controlled by: Liver meridian.
Element: Earth.
Assigned feelings: Being wanted/being rejected.
Qualities: Rationality, analysis, digestion, and/or their opposite counterparts.

The Lung Meridian

Just as the heart meridian is related to the universal rhythms and vibrations, among other things, the lung meridian connects the human being with the rhythms of the surrounding world on this level of existence. It ensures that there is a smooth, even complementary and mutually constructive interplay of vibrations and structures of the outer world on the one hand and the individual need for specific environmental rhythms and structures on the other hand. This function has extremely diverse effects on the entire human being. Sor-

row and grief that are more or less openly apparent always arise when this functional cycle is disrupted. This is because the fundamental needs of a human being, which can only be satisfied through contact with the outer world, tend to not be taken as seriously as they should be. Fanaticism and dogmatism of all types, as well as very distinct ideas of "what's good for all people" and how life should be, have their roots in an imbalance of this meridian. If the lung meridian is disrupted for a longer period of time, the respective person will be torn by increasingly intense despair without necessarily being able to come up with a concrete reason for feeling this way. Since he often no longer perceives his deeply human needs at this stage, he also cannot recognize the reason for his suffering.
Works together with: Large intestine.
Controlled by: Heart meridian.
Element: Metal.
Assigned feelings: Being cheerful/being depressed.
Qualities: Intuition, creativity and/or their opposite counterparts.

The Kidney Meridian

This meridian contains the physical and spiritually inherited predispositions. At the same time, the spleen meridian gives this functional cycle the experiences that the individual has acquired and that fit in with his plan for life to be stored and passed on to the physical and spiritual offspring, or for having it call up the appropriate experiences in order to be capable of employing them in a certain function and taking them into consideration. In this respect, the kidney meridian also corresponds to the memory. It's interesting to note that people generally have a better memory of their experiences that are closely linked with their plan in life, meaning those that are passed on by the spleen-pancreas meridian to the kidney meridian. Older people with a weakened spleen-pancreas function have a good memory of events that took place long ago since they are still stored in the kidney meridian. However, their short-term memory is often less intact since this is essentially organized through the spleen-pancreas meridian. Moreover, this functional cycle influences the flow of vital energy in general. All types of feelings that have been experienced, an uncramped posture and musculature, and the ability to adapt to the flow of life therefore indicate a harmonious energy relationship within the kidney meridian. Psychoses of all types are generally related to this meridian.

Works together with: Bladder meridian.
Controlled by: Spleen meridian.
Element: Water (This element symbolizes vital energy and feelings in many esoteric systems.)
Assigned feelings: Faithfulness/unfaithfulness, security/insecurity in relationships.
Qualities: Primal trust, faithfulness, tradition and/or their opposite counterparts.

The Circulation-Sex Meridian

The collection and release of joyful, pleasure-seeking energy is the task of the circulation-sex meridian. Restlessness, depression, feelings of oppression, angina pectoris, and other problems indicate a dysfunction here. The body lives out of joy. If a pleasurable lifestyle is limited by discipline and a falsely understood sense of duty, it's only natural for symptoms of reluctance to occur. On the other hand, an overemphasis on physical desire exhausts this energy reservoir. This meridian primarily influences the physical/functional activities.
Works together with: Triple warmer meridian.
Assigned feelings: Satisfied/worried.
Qualities: Desire/reluctance.

The Gallbladder Meridian

This meridian passes on the energies of the liver meridian and brings them to the outside. It's related to the ability to make decisions and therefore to health disorders that have their cause in a lack of decisiveness.
Works together with: Liver meridian.
Element: Wood.
Assigned feelings: Modesty/pride.
Qualities: Vitality, emotion, dynamism and/or their opposite counterparts.

The Small Intestine Meridian

This meridian is responsible for the absorption and transformation of all types of energies within the entire body. It also separates the energies beneficial for the body from those that are not, distributing the former to the areas where they are required and passing the others on to be eliminated.

Works together with: Heart meridian.
Element: Fire.
Assigned feelings: Being valued/not being valued.
Qualities: Joy, desire, love, unity and/or their opposite counterparts.

The Stomach Meridian

This meridian is the central "buffer" of the organism. All energetic impacts that the organism can't process are taken into this functional cycle so that the surplus doesn't cause any harm. If an energy is lacking somewhere in the body, it is then called up from the stomach meridian and made available to the area that needs it at the moment. The importance of its harmonizing effect is demonstrated in the rule of Chinese medicine that says no healing reaction can be initiated without a functioning stomach meridian. You experience the function of the meridian when, for example, you are frightened and this feeling first hits you in the stomach. It's better for the organism to let the stomach absorb such a shock than for the constant functioning of more important regulatory systems to be thrown off track by the concentrated charge of energy. If the stomach can't intercept an impulse, it continues on to the spleen meridian. If this is severely burdened, its antagonist—the kidney meridian—must greatly exert itself in order to reinstate equilibrium and can, if the impact is strong and sudden, be excessively strained. This may trigger kidney failure, which can lead to death if it isn't treated.
Works together with: Spleen meridian.
Element: Earth.
Assigned feelings: Reliable/unreliable.
Qualities: Rationality, analysis, digestion and/or their opposite counterparts.

The Large Intestine Meridian

This meridian participates in the transmission of all types of energies. Because of feelings of guilt, which are ultimately an act of holding onto oppressive energies, it can be disrupted. In such a case, further harmful energies are automatically clung to there, which can lead to a poisoning of the organism over time. This is why it's so important for physical and mental health, and for spiritual growth, to free yourself from self-poisoning/self-punishing through feelings

of guilt. A basic sadomasochistic attitude always has its roots in a disrupted large intestine meridian.
Works together with: Lung meridian.
Element: Metal.
Assigned feelings: Being compassionate/being embittered and guilty/innocent.
Qualities: Intuition, creativity and/or their opposite counterparts.

The Bladder Meridian

This meridian is responsible for keeping the body's energies in motion and, as a result, for relaxation in the broadest sense of the word. The master point of pain (acupuncture) is found on it, and it provides the spinal column with vital energy. The bladder meridian organizes the collection and timely release of special energies required for the functioning of the body. Disorders in this functional cycle become evident in the form of tensions, particularly in the area of the back, pain, and mental inflexibility. These disorders are usually caused by the fear of movement in the largest sense of the word.
Works together with: Kidney meridian.
Element: Water.
Assigned feelings: Patient-meaningful/impatient-meaningless.
Qualities: Primal trust, faithfulness, tradition and/or their opposite counterparts.

The Triple Warmer Meridian

Collections of energy within the body are created and dissolved through this meridian. It also serves to direct harmful energies out of the body and produces the connections of the functional cycles with each other. It therefore regulates the flow of overall vital energy in a certain respect. Pain, paralysis, and numbness are all related to functional disorders in the triple warmer.
Works together with: Circulation-sex meridian.
Assigned feelings: Willingness to help/humiliation
Qualities: Warmth/cold, full/empty.

The Conception Vessel

This meridian collects and regulates all the yin energies of the body. The conception meridian is also a reservoir for yin energies. In the

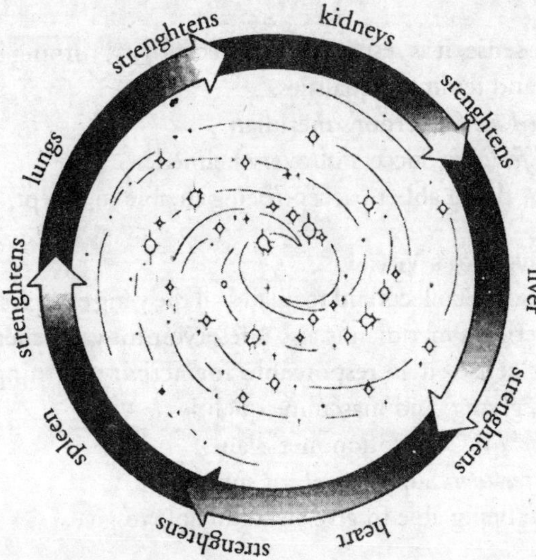

Constructive Meridian Cycle

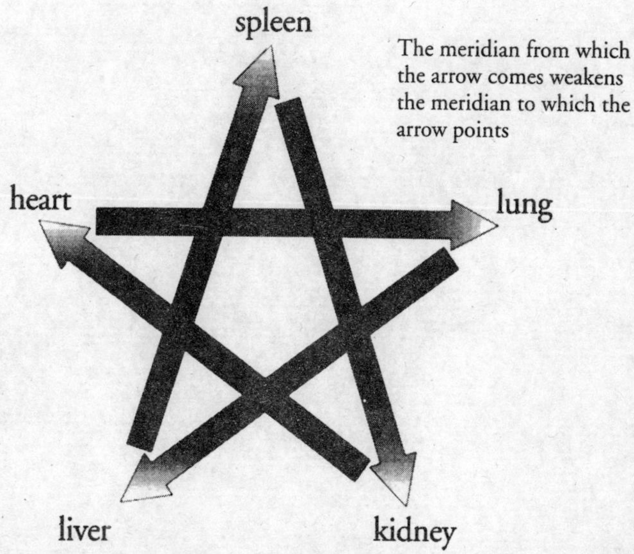

Weakening Meridian Cycle

broadest sense, it is responsible for receptivity, turning inwards, collection, and feminine qualities.
Controlled by: Governor's meridian.
Assigned feelings: Successful/overwhelmed.
Qualities: Being able to accept/being unable to accept.

The Governor's Vessel

This meridian collects and regulates all the yang energies of the body. The governor's meridian is also a reservoir for yang energies. In the broadest sense, it is responsible for activity, turning outwards, strength, giving, and masculine qualities.
Controlled by: Conception meridian.
Assigned feelings: Supportive/not supportive.
Qualities: Being able to give/being unable to give.

The Twelve Most Important Secondary Chakras

The next energetic level consists of the secondary chakras. There's an entire series of these. I've selected twelve of them with more comprehensive significance in reading auras for this description. In my experience, the secondary chakras can't be directly assigned specific colors. You will always perceive them in the colors of the main chakras with which they are connected at the time. These connections can change in accordance with current demands. A secondary chakra that tends to be separate from the main chakras will therefore show a pale color without any luminosity. If it is "stuck" in a connection, the coloration won't change even if the situation does. Always test in case of doubt.

The Yin and the Yang Chakra

These two important secondary chakras are located respectively at the center of the left shoulder (yin chakra) and the right shoulder (yang chakra), and they open upward. They fulfill a function similar to that of the much larger and more complicated crown chakra (seventh chakra) above the top of the head, yet are not nearly as comprehensive. They are both transmitters and receivers for the respectively associated portion of the body-mind-soul. Their development shows the realization of this part of the personality.

When fully developed, these two centers connect into an arc of light that runs behind the head when the respective person has learned to completely love and live both of these earthly (in the stricter sense) aspects, but hasn't yet achieved their unification with the more comprehensive consciousness of unity in love. Moments in which the first or even the second synthesis has been attained are among the great events in the life of a human being. Very few people succeed in the lasting realization of these energies. One method of promoting this and integrating the development harmoniously into everyday life without willfully forcing a certain orientation is the initiation MEDITATION OF THE THREE RAYS, which I teach.

Disorders in these chakras can, for example, be a lack of identification with an individual's own gender and problems in dealing with varying types of yin and/or yang energies. On the physical side, disorders can occur in the production of the sexual hormones.

These chakras are less developed in small children. At this stage, the seventh chakra still carries out the functions of the yin/yang chakra, which are vital for life. The more these two secondary chakras develop, the more the seventh chakra recedes in its dominating function for the time being. An essential step in the shifting of this function is puberty, and an even more profound step is the first completed sexual intercourse with a partner of the opposite sex.

Because of the tremendous energetic effects on the inner energy system, "innocent" children and babies, as well as virgin females and (less known) also virgin males, are attributed a substantial significance for certain rituals in the tradition of magic. This is because only energies that have not yet been strongly imprinted by yin and yang can be used to achieve specific effects. Since sorcerers generally have no access to the crown chakra because they lack loving acceptance of their own personality, they are dependent on an "energy swipe" for such exercises.

Traditional Tantra and special forms of Taoist Yoga develop these secondary chakras in a deep and lasting manner. However, the crown chakra must be indirectly included in the exercises after a certain stage. Otherwise, there could be a short-circuiting of the vital energy due to one-sided overloading.

The development of the yin/yang secondary chakras is among the fundamental tasks of earthly existence and is automatically and harmoniously done by all individuals who come to an expanded synthesis with the universal energy through loving acceptance of sexuality in everyday life over the course of time. But since this path is less spectacular and requires living sexuality in a loving way in the broadest sense, instead of turning away from it or transforming it, most people find it less attractive and therefore neglect it. The same can be said for many other natural paths of harmonious personality development in other areas.

The Nutrition/Responsibility Secondary Chakras

These two secondary chakras are located about two fingers beneath the two collarbones and open to the front. On the back side of the body, they are connected with the rest of the chakra energy system through curves of the ida and pingala main energy conductive pathways. They organize learning in long-term relationships by taking over tasks and, with respect to this, accepting what we experience on the basis of them (nutrition). Evidence of functional disorders is a cramped clinging to oppressive responsibility or fear of taking on responsibility. One additional, frequent functional disorder is the phenomenon of not being able to learn from the experiences we have had and therefore getting into the same situation over and over again.

These secondary chakras are closely related to the female breasts as organs of nutrition for infants, making them generally more distinct in women than men as energy centers. However, this isn't just a hereditary, but also an acquired quality.

The Elbow Chakras

There are secondary chakras in the area of all the joints. Many of them aren't very important for reading the aura. However, the elbow chakras have such a significant function that I've included them in the description. They are located a bit outside the respective tip of the elbow in the aura, yet still directly and closely connected with the body's inner energy field. Their tasks include acceptance and setting limits within a relationship, which means regulating its intensity.

Frequent disorders are therefore a lacking ability to set limits (can't say "no") and/or a too weakly developed ability to accept (can't say "yes"). Furthermore, inflexible and abrupt patterns of behavior when entering into relationships/contacts and setting limits against undesired relationships/contacts indicate a block of these chakras. Assertiveness, which means the pressure with which a person's own needs are fulfilled within relationships, is controlled through these centers. In the process, the left side regulates the emotional and the right side the intellect-related assertiveness.

The Palm Chakras

These energy centers are found in the palms of the hands and are connected with the outside world from there through the aura. They exchange information with the rest of the chakra system through the energy pathways at the backs of the hands. In addition, there are secondary chakras in the finger pads that are less significant within this context and basically have functions similar to those of the palm chakras, yet to a more limited extent.

The tasks of these secondary chakras include expressing the energies of all the chakras in relationships, as well as the perception of every type of subtle power that come close to the body from the outside. Blocks in these chakras can become evident in lacking sensitivity in relationships. A handshake that is too firm or too limp, cold hands, or blood congestion in these area can also be related to this theme. A lack of the ability to express oneself and have a "finely tuned" exchange with others, clumsiness, and too little artistic skill are other possible forms of expressing dysfunctions of these energy centers.

The Knee Chakras

These energy centers are located, similar to those of the elbow chakras, a bit above the knee-caps and are solidly linked to the inner energy system. They are connected with the other chakras at the hollow of the knee. They organize the ability to teach and learn in the broadest sense. Blocks may be expressed in the form of an overly critical attitude, constant skepticism, pride, arrogance, inferiority complexes, and megalomania.

A complete block of both knee chakras is linked with approaching death (life is learning!). Extensively developed knee chakras give the entire organism outstanding liveliness, strength, and flexibility, as well as protection against all the different kinds of blows of fate. A person who completely accepts teaching and learning (which are ultimately the same thing!), doesn't need to give himself any "broad hints" in order to finally look into a certain area of life and experience it.

The Sole Chakras

These energy centers are found at the center of the soles of the feet and are in contact with the outer world from this point. They are connected with the inner energy system from above the back of each foot. Just like the hands, the feet also have additional secondary chakras in each toe pad with similar functions but limited capacity. The sole chakras connect all other chakras with the earth. These receive the energies there that they need for healthy functioning and pass on to the ground the forces that they can't utilize.

The foot chakras basically have a similar function in relation to the earth as the hand chakras have in relation to living beings in the narrower sense. Defective functions can also be caused by working with the upper chakras at a point in time that is too early or do this too frequently, by too much meditation and meditation that is poorly guided, and by fear of the world because of all types of traumas. A lack of grounding, feelings of unreality, losing touch with reality, not paying attention to material/physical needs are some of the possible symptoms.

Fully functional sole chakras enable a harmonious development of spiritual qualities. Just like a tree needs healthy, strong roots in order to thrive well, a human being is dependent upon well-functioning foot chakras in order to be physically and emotionally/mentally healthy.

The Seven Main Chakras

These energy centers located on the center line of the body have a crucial significance for the regulation of the vital-energy processes on all levels. At the same time, they also represent the development of a human being in the area for which they are responsible.

In my system, the chakras one—six are divided into three groups: root (first) and sexual (second) chakra belong to the earth group, the solar plexus (third) and heart (fourth) chakra to the human being group, and the throat (fifth) and forehead (sixth) chakra to the heaven group. The energy centers one, three, and five essentially organize the yang energies (idea) and the centers two, four, and six the yin energies (experience).

When there are blocks in a yang chakra over a longer period of time, these always have an effect on the other yang chakras, usually in an upward direction. The same applies to the yin chakras.

The earth group looks after functions absolutely necessary for survival on the material level: survival through fight and flight, maintenance of the race through reproduction, the sensory contact to the world, and enjoyment of it are the basic preconditions for experiences and the exchange of energies.

The human being group is responsible for functions that are absolutely necessary for the development of the human form of existence: individualization, the ability to have relationships, the ability to analyze and project, as well as the ability to act as an individual in the sense of the group and still maintain a connection to the unity despite all the qualities of individuality.

The heaven group is responsible for functions that enable a person's spiritual development: resonance of being, communication on all levels, perceiving and following one's own, unique path in harmony with the structure of the Creation.

Assigning the chakras to the individual levels can save you much work in reading auras because you can quickly and assuredly find out how the individual areas' expression are related to each other. This makes it easier to recognize possible imbalances within the personality. In the ideal case, the lower levels are more strongly accentuated in energetic and structural terms than the upper levels since they must contribute the energy and stability to the human and/or spiritual development. This results in the chakra system having a

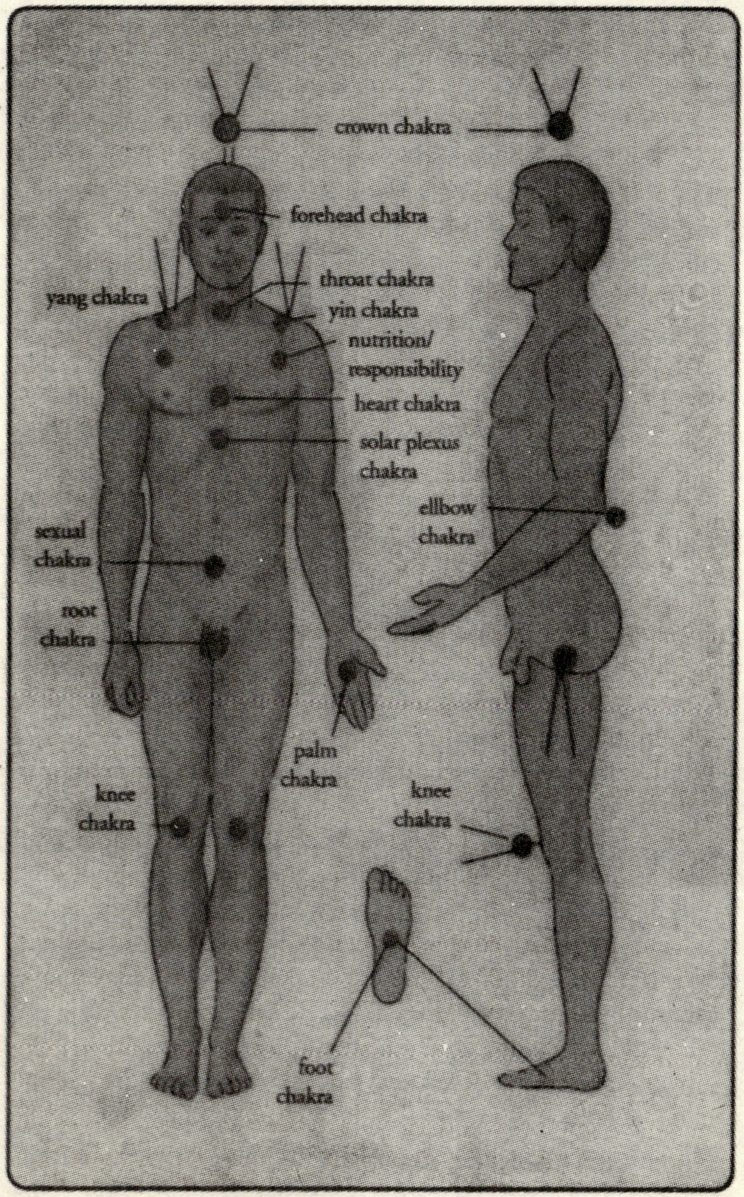

Main and Secondary Chakras

form like a pyramid: the more strongly developed centers are below and the weaker ones are on top. If the pyramid is standing on its head, meaning that the upper centers are distinctly more strongly developed than the lower ones, the perception, actions, and grounding of the personality will more or less be disturbed. If the chakra system tends to be structured like a spindle, meaning with a well-developed middle section but weakly developed upper and lower areas, this person will have difficulty in developing his potential in some sort of lasting manner. The power required to set something in motion is also lacking, as well as the ability of expressing who he is. His ability to have relationships is too weakly developed for him to be able to receive extensive support from other people. So, if he doesn't want to develop himself, he will only roam through life like a lonely wolf.

You can learn more about the chakra constellations by studying the I Ching. But first, here is a description of the main chakras.

The Root Chakra

Position: On the perineum between the vagina and the anus in the woman, between the scrotum and the anus in the man. It radiates into the aura toward the earth and is connected with the inner energy system through the coccyx.

Color: Red (In its ideal state, without yellow or blue components and tones of black or white!).

The will to exist on the material level is manifest in this energy center. The abilities of fighting and fleeing necessary for survival, as well as for the preservation of the species, are organized here. It has a structuring effect on all living processes. Frequently occurring disorders here are: exaggerated combat readiness (looking for risks!), exaggerated pacifism (everyone else should live, I'm glad to do without for their sake!), a lack of structure (disorder; confused talking, thinking, and acting; chaotic lifestyle), and too much structure (discipline, fulfillment of duties).

An excellent possibility for promoting the harmonious development of the root chakra is learning a martial art (judo, karate, Wing Chun, Kung Fu, Tai Chi Chuan, etc.) with an experienced, responsible teacher.

This energy center has a close relationship to the bones, nails, teeth, the vitality of the blood, and all long-lasting, chronic health disorders, as well as the ability to regenerate after stress. In addition, the legs and feet are closely connected with the first chakra (exchange with the earth, being rooted). The root chakra also has a direct link with the so-called limbic system, the part of the brain responsible for self-preservation (food, attack and defense) and the preservation of the species (sexuality).

The Sexual Chakra

Position: Just above the pubic bone at the center of the body. It radiates to the front into the aura and is attached to the inner energy system at the corresponding point on the spinal column.
Color: Orange (In the ideal state, equal parts of red and yellow, without any touches of black or white).

This energy center is responsible for the physical nature, the ability to encounter others, and the joy of living in the broadest sense. The perception of one's own body and the outside world on all levels and the enjoyment of these contacts is made possible here. This is why I prefer to call this center the relationship or love-of-life chakra instead of the sexual chakra. Although sexuality—in any case the lusty, relationship-supporting, harmonizing aspect of this energy—is at home in this chakra (the species-preserving aspect is subject to the first chakra), this only represents a small, partial aspect of the entire spectrum of this energy center's tasks. Frequent blocks are: a diminished love of life ("It's more important for me to do my duties, follow laws, etc. than to enjoy life!"); fear of closeness in any form; sexuality that is excessively emphasized ("Sex is the only thing that gives me the feeling of being alive!") or rejected ("I've risen above sex, I've transformed it, don't need it, it's something for animals, etc."); fear of heights, falling, and flying; sexual disorders of all kinds; a lacking or diminished body feeling.

The second chakra has a relationship to everything liquid within the body, to the organs that produce, process, and store fluids, to the hair and skin, and to the urogenital system in general. A further important connection exists with the limbic system, which is a part of the brain (for explanation: see under Root Chakra).

One effective method of harmoniously developing the second chakra is traditional(!) Tantra. More modern Western systems that call themselves Tantra aren't necessarily related to the original Tantra. Just as useful in this respect is the Gestalt Therapy founded by Perls and the Usui System of Reiki, a highly effective form of work with non-polar life energy, which anyone can learn easily.

The Solar Plexus Chakra

Position: One hand below the end of the breastbone at the center of the body. It radiates to the front into the aura and is connected at the same height on the spinal column with the inner energy system. *Color:* Yellow (In the ideal state, without any touches of blue and red and without black or white tones).

In this energy center, the ability to be an individual, to analyze and manipulate (power!) the energies and substances that come into a human being's range of influence is expressed. Without these abilities, neither digestion (mental/emotional and physical), nor conscious thinking, projecting, and analyzing is possible. The ability to set limits, to say "no," is also provided here. Frequent blocks are: fears, helplessness, feelings of guilt, karmic burdens*, lacking energetic presence (mousy person) or strong energetic pressure in the way a person acts (powerhouse).

This chakra has a relationship to all functions and organs of digestion, to the physical and mental ability to deal with stress, to being personally centered (inner peace, stability of personality), and to the nervous system. There is also a connection to the eyes as the analytical sense.

Methods for developing this chakra are psychoanalysis in its many forms, bioenergetics, Zen meditation, and inner martial arts like Tai Chi Chuan, Kai Sai, Kung Fu, Hsing I, Pa Kua, and Aikido.

---

* I understand karmic burdens not as God-intended punishment but as the refusal of an individual to let go of a relationship—which means to say "no"–or have a fair exchange in a relationship so that this creates neither an energy deficit in the one person (which is always connected with a feeling of duty or guilt toward the other) nor an excess of energy (which is always connected with a frequently unconscious claim to power toward the first person). This also includes so-called "selfless help," "just living for the sake of other person/a good purpose," in short–everything that is generally summed up by the term "helper syndrome." Also compare this with my description of the universal laws of energy exchange in *Reiki–Way of the Heart*, Lotus Light/Shangri-La.

The Heart Chakra

Position: One hand below the armpits at the center line of the body on the breastbone. It radiates to the front into the aura and is attached to the inner energy system exactly opposite on the spinal column.

Color: Green (In an ideal state, equal parts of yellow and blue without any black or white tones).

The heart center organizes the ability to accept the world as it is. In a certain sense, this chakra has crucial significance for a human being. If he doesn't learn to accept and love himself with his errors, weaknesses, and strengths (which are all basically the same!), he will more or less be sick, weak, and unhappy. No chakra can function properly and harmoniously if it isn't connected to the power of the heart center.

On the other hand, the heart chakra must have an energetic foundation and protection through a well-developed solar plexus chakra so that it doesn't become overtaxed. Only when I can say "no" do I also have the possibility of saying "yes." Human beings are not infinitely able to accept things and cannot achieve this state on this level of existence. We are here to learn how to love, and this only works when a person learns to deal with the errors and weaknesses of the world and with his self. When everything is perfect, no love is necessary.

The power of this center is also closely linked with the development of the second chakra. If I don't perceive myself and the world—or only do so through rose-colored glasses—then I can't learn to love things like they are: with everything that I don't like and which possibly even hurts me, and also with the things that I don't understand, the sense of which I don't want to or can't grasp.

Frequent blocks in the heart chakra are: dogmatism, fanaticism, glossing over things, black/white thinking (the white and black brotherhoods, God and the Devil, good and evil, good people and bad people/powers/opinions; creating hierarchies of all kinds; presumption; feelings of inferiority, etc.), and intolerance.

The attitude of "I love you because...!," "You must learn to love!," "The power of love/God/Jesus will do...for me!," "I fight with the powers of love against evil!," and the like is frequently declared as love but can actually be seen as something quite different and should instead be classified as functional disorders of the third chakra (claims to power). Love accepts without "if" and "but." It doesn't fight.

The heart chakra has a close relationship to the heart, the lungs, the ingesting part of the digestive system, particularly the small intestine, and the immune system (if I love myself, I protect myself!), and above all, the thymus gland. Furthermore, it is closely linked to subtle perceptions of all types (partially in cooperation with the second and the sixth chakra).

Methods for developing the heart chakra are the Usui System of Reiki, Aikido, I Ching work, and gestalt therapy, among others.

The Throat Chakra

Position: Three fingers below the larynx at the center line of the body. It radiates to the front into the aura and is attached to the inner energy system two fingers above the prominent cervical vertebra at the cervical vertebral column.
Color: Blue (In an ideal state, without any yellow and red mixed in and without black or white tones).

This energy center is responsible for self-expression and active communication on all levels. It is the chakra that enables us to artistically express our own personality (bringing inner beauty to the outside) and the formation of life habits and the body, as well as active manipulation of others.

In contrast to the third chakra's use of power, which is basically just aimed at separating the usable from the non-usable or restructuring and bringing together energies and substances so that the body can employ them for its maintenance and construction (which is an essentially passive application of the ability to manipulate), the fifth chakra can actively give everything that is open to influence the structure that corresponds to the inner demands, the self of a human being. This is how books(!), music, painting, and the like are shaped by means of this chakra.

The harmonious development of the throat energy center is closely linked with the development of the heart chakra's qualities. If my ability to love is developed, I won't push others up against the wall with my self-portrayal but harmonious complement, support, and thereby intensify the individual self-expression of others. This makes up the choir of the living Creation, which J. R. R. Tolkien, the author of *Lord of the Rings,* so impressively describes in his book *The Silmarillion.*

The energetic qualities of all other chakras are expressed through the throat center. Distinct signs of their characteristics are the voice, posture and body language, facial expressions, form of the body, etc.

Frequent blocks of this center are: a monotonous, constantly loud or quiet voice; always the same speech modulation; few overtones in the voice; and the tendency to become stuck in the same way of behaving and having the same health disorders. Furthermore, the claim of shaping the world to be like my image of it (magical thinking); the fear of showing myself as I am; always wanting to be in the foreground or wanting to stay in the background; channeling (not in every case, but very frequently); problems with the sense of hearing.

The fifth chakra has a strong relationship to the larynx and vocal chords, the skeleton, the skeletal musculature, the thyroid gland, the process of inhaling and exhaling, and the sense of hearing.

Methods for developing the throat chakra include singing overtones, the Alexander Technique, Tai Chi Chuan, art therapy, and artistic creativity of all types, pottery-making, free dance, belly-dance, bioenergetics, Reichian body work, and related methods.

The Forehead Chakra

Position: One finger above the line of the eyebrows at the center of the body. It radiates to the front into the aura and is attached to the inner energy system at the height of the medulla oblongata at the back of the head.

Color: Violet (In an ideal state, with equal parts of blue and red, without any black or white tones).

Through this energy center, also called the third eye, the spiritual ability of sensing and understanding one's own path, as well as sensing and understanding the path of the Creation in general, is made possible. This ability is also called intuition. Intuition should not be confused with feeling. As long as fear or greed are involved, intuition will not be capable of developing completely. For this reason, this chakra is also the last in the series of main chakras located within the body. Only when all the other energy centers are completely accepted, lived, and loved with their qualities can the third eye open harmoniously—the personal path has then been accepted and followed in connection with the development of the universe.

Frequent blocks of the sixth chakra are: instability (not finding one's own path, one's own way of living); visions, premonitions, and "seeing ghosts"; orienting one's lifestyle according to a guru, master, or some sort of behavior pattern provided by the outside world; feeling that one's own life is futile; no relationship to God (no matter what name we use here).

There is a close relationship of the sixth chakra to the eyes, the understanding function of consciousness (understanding = bringing together analytic and synthetic thinking into a holistic perspective). If you are taken aback here: I consider synthetic thinking not to be holistic but as a meaningful and necessary complement to analytic thought. Here's a thought-provoking impulse: Neither the analytically acquired computer-image calculations nor the hologram are actually the landscape. Further connections: pituitary gland and pineal gland (tends toward the latter the more the third eye is accepted).

Methods for developing the sixth chakra include the Usui System of Reiki (starting with the Second Degree), decade work, dyads, work with the I Ching and Tarot, and gestalt therapy.

The Crown Chakra

Position: Three fingers above the top of the head*. The seventh chakra is connected with the inner energy systems through the master point on top of the head. Radiates in all directions.

Color: White (all colors). In the ideal state, all colors are equally represented. This means that you could theoretically get all the important information about the state of a person's chakras by reading the crown chakra. However, this often doesn't work in the practice because of the abundance of patterns and colors in this energy center.

The seventh chakra, also called the crown chakra, is the expression of the universal unity consciousness and the unification of opposites on all the levels of a human being. It behaves in a passive way

---

* You can discover the position of your crown chakra by doing the following little exercise: Place the front area of the index finger and middle finger of one hand precisely above the top of the head in a vertical position. Now feel into your body. If you can clearly perceive your physical condition, then also move your middle finger above the other two. Now feel into your body again and pay attention to the changes. Don't hold your fingers above the top of your head too long and only do this perceptive exercise infrequently. Some people get a headache from it!

until the respective person has learned to adequately love and live the qualities of the lower six chakras. Then it begins to be active and make the body-mind-soul into a direct expression of the divine energy. Then God, human being, and universe are one, although they are separate. In general, people in this state either retreat to another level of existence in order to prepare new possibilities of experience or they remain on the earth and are only active in the background and on specific occasions. These people have nothing to do with the described spiritual hierarchies or masters of the world.

Hierarchies are connected with the development of the third and fifth chakra or with their functional disorders. For people with a developed third eye and crown chakra, a place within a hierarchy is a step backward in their evolution.

Frequent blocks: See chakras one to six.

Methods for harmonious development of this chakra: See chakras one to six.

The Various Functional Levels of the Main Chakras

In order to better understand the main chakras' great diversity of tasks, it's helpful to know something more about their functional level. Chakras are frequently defined in a very one-dimensional way today. But they aren't one dimensional. In addition to classifying their general areas of activity, it can also be determined that they have different temporal levels, which in turn are penetrated by further subtle/energetic levels. There is also a functional level that crosses all the others and is responsible for feedback with the material body, as well as for the karmic levels. According to the relative charging (for explanation, see below), these karmic levels also influence certain other levels. I will outline the essential levels in the following. CL stands for chakra level.

Time-Oriented Functional Levels

The level of the spiritual predispositions (CL 1):

The fundamental spiritual constitution of a human being is stored here. Truly intensive experiences of this type are also stored here and passed on to spiritual students (we all have some of these in the course of our lives!) and kept for later incarnations. There are connections to the various levels of racial memory in certain cases.

The level of the predispositions inherited through the family (CL 2):

Here are all types of predispositions inherited from the physical predecessors. When intensive processes take place within a human being, new things are additionally stored or old things are changed.

The level of the acquired predispositions (embodied) (CL 3):

These are the abilities and all types of solidly integrated patterns of behavior acquired during the course of a lifetime. Information from this area can be passed on to the chakra levels 1 and 2 under certain circumstances.

The level of the acquired predispositions (non-embodied). (CL 4):

Acquired abilities and patterns of behavior that can be cast aside again (forgotten) in a relatively easy manner. Under certain preconditions, these contents are passed on to the chakra level 3.

The level of the main learning line for one incarnation cycle (CL 5):

(The main learning lines are differentiated in the individual chakras only through certain focal points, which correspond to the functional area of an energy center. Otherwise, they are the same in all the chakras and connected with each other as well).

These are the areas of experience that you have chosen for a number of lives, but not necessarily in their consecutive order. Don't confuse this with karma! This also applies to the subsequent levels of the learning lines.

The level of the main learning lines of an incarnation (CL 6):

These are the areas of experience that you have chosen for one lifetime. Whether you will become a beggar or a bank director isn't stored here. The shaping of the learning situation is largely up to your momentary freedom to make decisions and can also be influenced within this scope by the actions of other participants in the great game of life. This tends to apply more when you reject personal responsibility for the shape of your life and less when you accept this responsibility. This also is valid in accordance with the other learning lines.

The level of medium-term main learning lines (CL 7):

These are the areas of experience that you have chosen for certain related areas of a lifetime, which are frequently cycles of 10, 7, or 6 years.

The level of the short-term main learning lines (CL 8):

These are the areas of experience that you have chosen for periods of time that are relatively easy to keep track of, frequently ranging from a few months to a year.

The level of the momentary events (CL 9):

All of the events taking place at the current moment are reflected in this layer, as well as the organization of the processes on every level necessary for this purpose. This level can also be further subdivided, but I won't do this because it would take too much space. However, you should be able to work this out on your own by now.

Subtle/Energetic Functional Level

The level of the etheric body (CL 10):

This level connects all the other levels of a chakra with the etheric body, which is a component of the aura. For the description, see further below.

The level of the emotional body (CL 11):

This level connects all the other levels of a chakra with the emotional body, which is a component of the aura. For the description, see further below.

The level of the mental body (CL 12):

This level connects all the other levels of a chakra with the mental body, which is a component of the aura. For the description, see further below.

The level of the spiritual body (CL 13):

This level connections all the other levels of a chakra with the spiritual body, which is a component of the aura. For the description, see further below.

Level of Body Feedback (CL 14)
This level connects all the other levels of a chakra with the body. This means that energetic changes on all levels within the body can be expressed on the one hand, and changes of the body in the respective chakra levels can be registered and taken into consideration in the organization of vital energetic processes on the other hand. This level can naturally be further subdivided (material body in the narrower sense, meaning everything that can be touched; material body in the broader sense, meaning meridians, reflex zones, energetic organ functions, and secondary chakras).

Individual Karma Level (CL 15)
This is the level where you hold onto certain relationships and therefore deny yourself of possibilities for development. Resolving karma is relatively easy here. There are direct connections to the fields of the aura.

Social Karma Level (CL 16)
This level supplements the previous one with relationships of large groups, of which you are a part, that haven't yet been released. Resolving this karma is more difficult than in CL 15. There are connections to the fields of the aura.

Race Karma Level (CL 17)
This level supplements the previous two with relationships of the race "human being" that haven't yet been released. Resolving this karma is very difficult for the individual.* There are connections to the fields of the aura.

The latter three levels can also be further subdivided.

As an aside, karma doesn't just have negative aspects, but also very positive ones. Take a close look at both sides and try to understand them. I'm not permitted to delve any deeper into this here.

---

* Extensive areas of these levels are harmonized in the Reiki initiations of the individual grades.

The Main Energy Channels Sushumna, Ida, and Pingala

These conductive pathways runs along (ida and pingala) the spinal column or in (sushumna) the spinal column from the pelvis to the head and connect all the main chakras and many of the secondary chakras directly, as well as indirectly connecting all other parts of the energy system with each other. This connection is particularly significant for the root chakra and the third eye since energies from the pelvic region are set into motion directly here at the demand of the forehead center. Blocks in these channels therefore have serious effects in all parts of the body-mind-soul. I have always discovered such a block in people who essentially hand over the responsibility for how they live their lives to someone else. The cause for this can be an overly intensive attachment to a teacher, guru, an oracle system—including astrology—or an ideology that establishes how a person lives in the place of taking personal responsibility for one's own life.

When an adequate state of personal development has been achieved, the so-called kundalini force, a very strong form of polar life energy stored in the root chakra in the coccyx, rises through the three energy channels to the crown chakra (seventh main chakra, located just above the top of the head). This gives the respective person great strength, facilitates access to the subtle abilities, but also represents one of the biggest challenges of the spiritual path with respect to the proper approach to personal power.

The Aura and the Four Subtle Bodies

In esotericism, the aura is understood to be a subtle energy field existing around the human body and consisting of a number of layers. It is formed to a minor degree by the emanations of the body's inner energy system. The other parts of the aura exist independently, even though they are generally connected as closely as possible with the material body. The existence of the aura can be indirectly proved with modern scientific means (Kirlian photography, Kilner-screen goggles). In the esoteric tradition, people have been aware of this phenomenon for thousands of years.

For our purposes, this energy field is very interesting since much detail work can be saved by observing and systematically evaluating it. Despite this, we comprehend the human being as a unity. If you are already familiar with reading and interpreting this energy field, your understanding of the other person will be intensified in a significant and simple way. When you give a reading, you therefore don't need to take such a detailed look around in other energetic areas in order to come to a meaningful and deep interpretation.

The aura consists of many, partially overlapping, individual fields. To keep this description from becoming too complicated, I will limit myself to the most important ones. In the context of reading and interpreting the other levels, this description is completely adequate in order to work well with it. The aura basically flows from the top of the head to the hands and—mainly—to the feet, meaning the earth. In the middle of the palms of the hands and the soles of the feet, the aura energy enters the body once again, after it has released the energetic patterns that the organism no longer needs or wants to express to the surrounding world. It then flows through special energy channels up to the top of the head, where it streams out like a fountain and begins the cycle of purifying powers anew. Through the flow of the aura energy, forces that the body no longer needs or that harm it, among other things, are passed on to the surrounding world, primarily to the earth.

In a certain sense, this energy field fulfills a function on the subtle level similar to that of the skin on the material level. It also participates substantially in the communication processes and uses its power to protect the inner energy system from the influence of environmental energies that are too strong or harmful.

The communication processes of the inner energy system can also run through the aura. Certain connections among the chakras are only possible in this way and other connections are activated when the internal lines of communication are obstructed for some reason. If the flow of the aura is disrupted—which can be seen during readings by whirls, dark spots, bands, and the like—the lines of communication located there and the energetic detoxification of the body no longer function properly. Poor grounding and a strong susceptibility to emotional/mental strains may have their cause here since the contact with the earth tends to be weakened. In this case, it's impossible to adequately pass on the surplus of energies and inharmonious forces that no longer can be processed to the ground. Depending on what forces these are, this may result in certain fields of the aura being affected as well since these must buffer undesired energies and be capable of slowly releasing them through different paths. This can lead to an intensely imbalanced personal magnetism, although the person can't do anything about it. This case often occurs after someone has spent a longer period of time with inharmonious people or stayed at places with difficult energy.

Draining off the entrenched forces can provide quick relief. If the aura can't completely buffer the inharmonious energies, the solar plexus chakra is burdened by them, which can possibly have recuperations on the corresponding meridians and subtle organ functions as well. Pay careful attention to such correlations when you do readings!

Three further time-related levels of the aura are also important for our purposes: the current, medium-term, and long-term levels, which permeate all four main fields of the aura. With the help of your Inner Child, you can separate them just like the other aura fields by asking it to show you or emphasize just the parts you desire to see. Read more about this in the next chapter. On the present-time levels of the aura, the energies currently in the foreground of shaping the life are depicted by one or more colors. You can associate these with the color classification of the chakras and interpret them within the context of the overall system.

When it is harmonious, this level is related to the short-term main learning lines in the chakras. The medium-term aura level shows the energies at the foreground of shaping the life for a longer period of time. When they are harmonious, there is a relationship to the medium-term main learning lines of the chakra level.

The long-term aura level shows the energies that are in the foreground of shaping the life in the long run. When they are harmonious, there is a relationship to the main learning lines of the incarnation on the chakra level. When these three levels are connected with each other through energy flows, this is generally a good sign. Similar colors or those which fit together well on the three time-related aura levels are also an expression of harmony.

Since the aura is a communication organ, energies that haven't been completely expressed to the surrounding world can also be observed within it. These are messages that have stayed on the tip of the tongue, so to speak. This intermediate storage function of the aura is very important since it isn't possible to express everything at any given time. The energy that is firmly held there only becomes a problem when it cannot be released at all. Then the aura is in a state of being overcharged with old impressions such as an excessively intensive fixation on the past, along with a reduced ability to perceive the present environment. Like a layer of cotton wool, the echoes of past experiences come between the body and the outside world, the here and now.

A specific clarification of the aura fields, conversations and exercises that direct attention to the here and now over and over again can help in such cases. Severe traumas can leave tears, a type of energetic scars, in the structure of the aura when the ability to perceive and intermediately store unpleasant impressions suddenly and drastically becomes overtaxed. If the disruptions are in the area of chakras, they will have particularly inharmonious effects. Here it is necessary to cautiously treat the injuries suffered and work on regenerating the aura fields by means of subtle energy work time and again. This healing process requires quite a bit of time and patience since the affected person will generally be very much afraid of touching the traumatized structures.

The Structure of the Aura's Energy Bodies

The Etheric Body

This portion of the aura is formed anew with every incarnation and contains the physical structure of the respective individual, his current and fundamental access to the universal life energy* in this life, in addition to his ability to intuit and take action on the subtle/energetic levels, meaning extrasensory perceptions and magic in the broadest sense. The etheric body is formed relatively close around the material body. How far it extends changes with the respective

* Within this context, I understand the universal life energy to be a non-polar energy form that organizes the correct use of all other vital forces in the holistic sense. It is the quality of life energy closest to the divine creative force in our material world.

vital condition of a person and his momentary access to the universal life energy. The size, shape, coloration, and thickness accordingly reveals much about a person's general state of health.

If it hasn't yet been possible to work through certain experiences of a previous lifetime and harmoniously integrate them into the personality, or if the respective person has clung to certain personal bonds and experiences after his death instead of releasing them and thereby being able to go into a new life with completely new prerequisites, or when someone has a task that spans more than one incarnation (for example, when he has made a Bodhisatt vow or was the grand master of a spiritual tradition that has died out), the corresponding patterns follow the karmic laws in flowing into the formation of a new etheric body as the child grows in the womb.

The etheric body is closely associated with the muscle armor rings and generally connected with the musculature of the material body. This is why related disruptions, similar to problems like lacking physical means of expression, are exhibited in it by one-sided, mask-like body language. The etheric body is therefore a type of double for the material body. People who unknowingly cause the poltergeist phenomenon have a continual overcharging of this aura field. In such cases, if help is provided in finding a pleasant physical activity, this overcharging is usually quickly reduced. Fear of physical closeness and the traumas related to it show up in this aura field as white areas. A strong need for physical affection, tenderness, a sense of security, and being held that is difficult to express is shown here in the form of black and/or orange.

When a human being develops from an embryo into an adult, the etheric body and the spiritual body first come into existence. The emotional body and mental body are formed with their help and through the confrontation with the surrounding world.

The Emotional Body

This field of the aura is independent to a large extent. It supports and organizes our emotional life and our instincts. Emotional energy that isn't lived out can manifest itself after a longer period of time or in greater charges in this portion of the aura as blocks (whirls, rings, etc.). The emotional body overlaps in part the etheric body, but is generally larger than the latter in how far it extends. When a person resorts to the instincts or stores unlived feelings, usually caused by fear or trauma or (seldom) consciously for magical purposes, it can extend very far. Some spiritual teachers consciously make use of the extension of the emotional body by charging it with certain emotional energies as a means of gaining access to other people and more easily conveying certain experiences to them. If this charging is done by individuals who haven't yet profoundly accepted themselves, it is then linked to great health risks. Even other people who are within this field can also suffer more or less intensive health impairments. So please don't experiment with this and pay attention to disproportionately extended emotional bodies when reading your client's aura in order to help him in this respect. The size of the emotional body and its changes during a conversation says a great deal about the strength of the emotional life that is permitted and maintained, as well as about the suppression of specific feelings. I often use a resonance test that I've developed for this purpose: During the conversation, I weave in terms like love, death, fear, sympathy, sorrow, sex, eroticism, intimacy, relationship, anger, aggression, hate, envy, etc. and make a note of how this part of the aura reacts shortly thereafter: a "0" for no substantial change, a "+" when it becomes larger, a "++" for much larger, a "–" for smaller, and a "– –" for much smaller. There may also frequently be changes in the form of the emotional body during this test. They can give information about that region of the body in which the affected emotions are blocked or expressed particularly well. Another test is to suggest that your client think of a certain emotion, then read his aura and make a note of your observations while he does so.

The coloration of the emotional body says a great deal about the emotional energies that stand in the foreground at the moment. A test similar to the one described above can be performed for this purpose. Clarity tends to indicate a good emotional flow, but a strong dark coloration tends to indicate stuck emotional energies (can sometimes also be observed above specific body zones!) or those that are very turbulent at the moment. During the healing process, the emotional body is often quite chaotic to look at. Be sure not to confuse this state with an emotional life that is actually inharmonious! After a certain start-up phase, you can observe forms and images in this part of the aura. They can usually be classified with one of the chakras or some other part of the energy system on the basis of their position, coloration, or meaning. They give information about feelings or triggers for them that are suppressed or strongly in the foreground. This is important for the deeper, practical interpretation of the chakra reading.

The Mental Body

The mental body organizes and supports all the thinking processes: both in the conscious and the unconscious sense, as well as partially or completely automatized patterns and processes of thinking and acting. Reflexes, valuations, ethical and moral ideals and dogmas are therefore at home in this area. The perceptions of the physical senses also flow into here and are processed and passed on in a partially conscious, partially unconscious manner. The mental body can penetrate both of the first two fields of the aura mentioned above, especially when the respective person places too much emphasis on the mental level. This doesn't mean that this person is highly intelligent or logical when it comes to evaluating impressions from the surrounding world, but just that he prefers the factual manner of processing information. A great deal of positive thinking, work with affirmations, and self-hypnosis can also produce or promote such a state*.

Otherwise, the mental body is located outside the emotional body. It can extend very far for hypnotists and people who live intensely from claims of power. If it overlaps the other bodies, the respective parts of the aura will then be dominated by it. When doing readings, please check to see whether this isn't just a momentary state! However, a certain penetration of the emotional body is healthy since this is evidence of the connection between the "mind and the belly."

If there is a clear line of separation between the mental and the emotional body, this can indicate a schizoid condition. Clear images in the mental body tell you much about the conscious and unconscious patterns of thought and imagination in the respective person. Their color makes it easier for you to assign them to a specific chakra. This can also be read with particular clarity if you do a resonance test. Say some catchwords that are related to the questions your client has asked and you will frequently see specific images in the mental body representing a distinct pattern. If the meaning of an image isn't clear to you, go ahead and ask because the person you are

* In such cases, be sure to always pay special attention to the solar plexus chakra and sexual chakra, as well as to the energetic state of the spleen!

talking to often knows the meaning. If not, do a chakra-reading on this symbol with the I Ching and let yourself be advised by a good version of the Book of Changes in terms of the interpretation.

All factual information that can't be completely expressed at the moment or that is to be taken into the inner energy system for evaluation is also stored in an intermediate manner in the mental body.

The Spiritual Body

A human being is connected with the divine plane, the level of unity, through this field of the aura. This is where certain subtle information is also received or transmitted. In contrast to the etheric body, which is also extensively involved with subtle energies, this deals particularly with transpersonal perceptions and actions. The spiritual body has a direct relationship to the crown chakra and to the heart chakra. It can overlap the other fields, particularly the latter two mentioned above, in people who have lovingly accepted themselves to a large extent, but normally extends further outward from the mental body. If a person is profoundly afraid of unification (examine the state of the sexual chakra for blocks!), the spiritual body can appear to be spatially separated from the other bodies. Then congestion and blocks in the emotional body and mental body can also usually be discovered, and the vital force (extension and radiant power of the etheric body) appears minimal.

The presence of people who have accepted themselves, Reiki initiations, experiences of enlightenment (in general or even of the individual chakras), and the like can increase the radiant power, position, and extension of the spiritual body for a more or less greater length of time. If you determine that the person has a well-developed spiritual body, precisely examine the condition of the other three fields of the aura and its correlation with it. If they are not as well-developed and don't have a transparent, powerful, and harmonious coloration, the current state of the spiritual body is not lasting. Nevertheless, one of the development-promoting patterns determined by the experiences mentioned in the previous text can anchor itself in the spiritual body so that, despite its long-term positive influence, it isn't perceptible in how the spiritual body develops. These patterns are quite powerful, yet so subtle that very few clairvoyants can observe and interpret them.

A very extensive spiritual body that still remains separate from the other fields of the aura indicates that a (great) talent as a teacher in life, guru (in the positive sense), holistic therapist, and the like, has yet to be integrated. During the development of the human being from embryo to adult, important integrated (and therefore not karmically active) experiences and perceptions are transferred to the other fields of the aura through the spiritual body.

The Relationship Between the Individual Life Levels

Your head is probably buzzing by now after working your way through this chapter. But it really isn't all that complicated. When doing a reading, you definitely don't need to take all the levels and correlations into consideration and know them by heart. This sketch of the vital energy system has been presented as extensively as possible in this book so that you can begin your readings with the area that is most easily accessible to you and have the necessary background information for a meaningful interpretation. Each individual has his own areas of the energy levels that he can better access in terms of perception and differentiation than another person. Find yours (how to do this is described in the following chapter) and work with it. With time and actual practice, the other levels will gradually open up to you totally on their own.

In order to round off this survey, I would like to describe in brief some important relationships between the levels:

It's only possible for the system of the muscle armor rings to exist largely independent of the normally existing control through the energetic main organs, meridians, and chakras when it is filled in part or completely with blocked energies. In this case, it's generally not possible to dissolve this type of congestion through the higher energetic levels. Direct bodily manipulation or medications that are effective on the basis of substances must be used. The muscle armor rings are normally controlled according to need through the superordinate levels. This system applies accordingly to all material components of the body.

The energetic main organs are the connecting links between the material and the energetic level. They control certain process quite autonomously. However, as long as they aren't energetically overloaded or totally empty, they are controlled and used generally in their function by the chakras and fields of the aura with respect to the integration in the overall system.

The main meridians are the connecting links between the higher and the lower energetic levels of the organism. If they are neither intensely overloaded nor empty, then they convey information and serve as intermediate storage areas, transmitters, and receivers for specific energy qualities.

The secondary chakras are essentially specialized field agencies for the various main chakras. Although they have a certain character of their own, they are essentially just responsible for certain areas of the body or narrowly limited task areas, thereby relieving the main chakras so that they aren't as quickly overloaded when a region is intensely strained on the one hand; on the other hand, they serve to carry the energy reserves that are called up when one chakra or one of the energetic main organs must emanate a great deal of power. In addition, they can catch energies coming into their region and pass them on to the rest of the inner energy system or the fields of the aura in small portions.

The main chakras are something like the senior head of a department in a large company. All the different lines of communication from all the areas of the body come together in them. In accordance with this, the state of the entire body is reflected in them. The chakras react to this information under consideration of the relative charge* of their individual levels and thereby control the processes of the overall organism.

---

* The relative charge of a chakra level, in my opinion, is the result of multiplying the amount of energy stored in this level and the event tension of this force in relation to the relative charges of the other chakra levels. The amount results from the energies that have reached this level from either the outside or inside, which are stored there for an intermediate period of time until they are called up. The event tension is a piece of information about the necessity of mobilization (motivation) of an energy stored in a level for mastering certain tasks of the body-mind-soul. In order to make this more vivid: Imagine that your digestive system isn't all that healthy and you should just eat small amounts of food at each meal and not too many meals a day because of this. However, your organism absolutely

Furthermore, the chakras bear various imprints in order to promote specific experiential situations (main learning lines). If the corresponding experiential situations are accepted and lived out, the energy existing in the main learning lines isn't blocked and therefore contributes to the better functioning of the overall organism. When these experiential situations are accepted and lived out to a large extent, this is felt to be an "opening" of the corresponding chakras or even as small act of enlightenment. This feeling has nothing to do with perceptions of flowing, streaming, or warming of body-energy work in the area of the lower energetic levels, which are frequently confused with a functional expansion ("opening") of the respective chakra. Chakras cannot be lastingly developed through physical manipulation, breathing exercises, visualizations, or any kind of meditative methods, energy transmission, or any type of medication but only as a result of living in a way that corresponds to the main learning lines and the loving acceptance of the experiences had as a result.

Exercises, medications, and energy transferrals, etc. can support and facilitate accepting and living the area of experience represented by a chakra up to a certain point, but never replace it. These processes don't have to take place in a conscious way; even experiences that aren't directly registered and prompted by the conscious mind fulfill this purpose if they are accepted by the subconscious mind.

The fields of this area are a human being's highest energetic region. They also reflect our overall state. In addition, they also carry important information of direct importance for the current incarnation and (with the exception of the etheric body, apart from special cases) also for the previous incarnations. They are additionally in contact with all the energies of the surrounding world. If the first three fields of the aura are too weakly expressed, every energetic

---

needs a mineral that it can only get in the necessary amounts when you frequently eat food in larger amounts in order to take care of a short-term task. You will then have an inclination of eating too much and too often, although this causes you digestive disorders and is unhealthy in the long run. The energetic power of the responsible levels in the third chakra is not high enough (low ability to digest = low amount of energy), but the need for the mineral is so great (strong motivation = high event tension) so that the process of energy release is initiated despite this. When the responsible storage area is empty, the reserves of other energy organs are used (tiredness after eating and digestive disorders because of using not completely compatible energy qualities from other levels).

contact will tend to be experienced as an infringement (often occurs when meditation practice is exaggerated or done with the wrong instructions!). When the aura fields are strongly charged (doesn't apply to the spiritual body), the energetic sensitivity is sometimes reduced to a state of numbness in this area (frequently happens when marital arts training is done with the wrong instructions, in very dogmatic people, and after intense states of shock, and can also effect partial areas).

Overview and Summary

Get acquainted with the energy system time and again. Don't learn it by heart, but try to comprehend it in practical terms in the form of little essays with examples from your own life. If you would like to get more deeply into this area, read books with more details about it and go to seminars on these topics.

First try to understand the system of the main chakras and the aura fields. When doing so, take into consideration that blocks always occur as a result of not wanting to live a quality and can only be eliminated in the long term by accepting and loving this quality. The stronger the block is, the more the other parts of the organism have demands placed on them so that they can provide the substitute functions, encapsulation energies, and counteractive forces in order to maintain the overall equilibrium. Chronic diseases are always sustained by this type of enormous expenditure of strength over a longer period of time. This interplay is particularly interesting in the area of the chakra levels.

Don't get stuck on the details but try to understand the overall system. In the appendix of this book you will find some pendulum tables that you should make additional use of, particularly when you first start reading auras in order to work out the finer points, main emphasis, and correlations. If you are familiar with an oracle system, you should additionally determine the themes of the individual areas by asking it. With time this will give you a very round picture of the overall system. The Tarot, I Ching, OH cards (a special oracle consisting of word and picture cards and dealing with emotions), Cards of Power, and naturally the excellent system of astrology are well-suited for this purpose. Runes are also appropriate. You should always check far-reaching interpretations with oracles when starting out, but not with the pendulum since it can be too easily influenced. The pendulum should support you in the reading, but not guide you in it.

Always(!) hold yourself back from valuations of what is moral and good/bad. The universe in its parts is neither good nor bad and not even shaped according to human morals, which constantly change anyway according to the place and time involved. It is. And this is how God wanted it because it would have been created it differently otherwise.

Now you should be adequately prepared for the next important step in learning to read the aura. In the following chapter we will look into how to work out the individual levels in a reading.

Chapter 5

Fine Tuning—Learning to Switch Between the Individual Levels of the Energy System

Now that we have sufficiently (I hope, in any case) looked into the energy system, the question inevitably arises as to how we can differentiate between these individual levels in a reading. In Chapter 4 you have already extensively worked your way into the practice of reading auras, more aptly called reading energy fields, but without knowledge about their many areas.

The easiest way to switch between the individual levels is to ask your Inner Child for help using its abilities in the subtle area. In the course of the following exercise, you can make an agreement with it to always show you exactly the areas that you want to see; and so that you have a good possibility of determining the energy qualities contained within them. It's really this simple. However, you should already know which area this is and what exactly you mean with this level. You should therefore thoroughly study the previous chapter and make it comprehensible for yourself in practical terms. This isn't a matter of "the only correct understanding" but of getting a clear picture at all. So don't worry about this. Simply look into the topics of the last chapter, then you will gradually but unavoidably grow in your(!) understanding of the levels and become clear about them. This is what it's all about.

So, now on to the exercise:

Relax by laying down comfortably, closing your eyes, and paying attention to your breathing. After a while, when your breath calmly and evenly flows in and out, briefly tense the muscle groups of your body tightly and then let go of them again right away. Next, ask your Inner Child to come into contact with you. When you receive a distinct sign of its attention, then greet it and tell it your wishes in clear and simple words. When you do a reading, ask it to show you the separate individual levels of the energy system that the two of you got to know extensively in the last chapter and respond to your desire of seeing a specific level. Don't give it orders but request it to do this and pay attention to see if it has reservations. If yes, then confront these in a fair and serious way and clear away the reasons for them. If you don't do this, your Inner Child won't work reliably with you. As a part of your self, by the way, it also has the right to be loved and have its wishes and reservations taken into consideration. If you open up to this, it will work with you willingly and well. In closing, thank it and tell it to inform you when it doesn't have any desire to do a reading. Then promise not to try to do it anyway but postpone it to another point in time. Absolutely keep this promise and, if possible, look into your inner partner's reasons for not wanting to do a reading at a certain point in time. This is very important for the development of your cooperation and your overall personality. You may often also receive surprising insights as a result.

For example, my Inner Child once strictly refused to carry out a reading that had long been scheduled for an acquaintance. Afterward, I discovered that an eclipse of the moon had taken place at this point in time, which would have totally falsified the result of the reading. So take your Inner Child seriously. It often knows more than you do and is more holistically concerned about your interests than the conscious portion of you since it receives a great deal of direct information from the surrounding world and—sometimes—from your Higher Self with its subtle senses.

If you want to make a further agreement about the depiction of subtle perceptions with your Inner Child, you can at any time make contact with it in the manner described above.

Practice switching between the individual levels after you have discussed all the necessary things with your Inner Child and written this down so that you can remember everything in exact detail later.

Do the extensive exercises discussed in Chapter 3 for perceiving the energy system; but this time, always do them so that you let your Inner Child show you a specific level. Once again note your observations on a copy of the body sketch that you have already used for the exercises in Chapter 3. Afterward, focus on the interpretation of your observations based on the information from Chapter 4. Write a brief, coherent text on the interpretation so that you get used to combining the individual observations and interpretations into a cohesive, meaningful, and succinct overall statement. It really takes frequent and serious practice to do this. When you can perform readings of the individual levels for yourself in a more or less certain

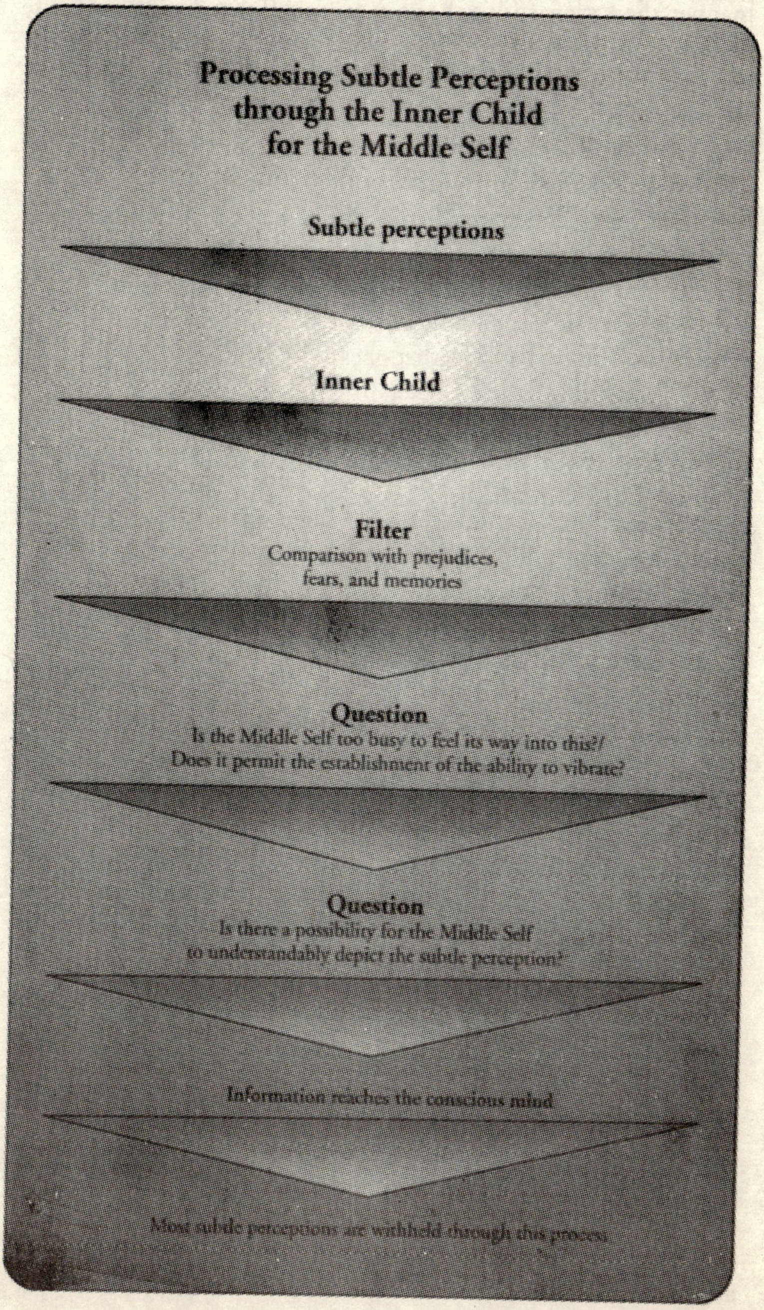

Processing Subtle Perceptions through the Inner Child for the Middle Self
Subtle perceptions
Inner Child
Filter
Comparison with prejudices, fears, and memories
Question
Is the Middle Self too busy to feel its way into this?/
Does it permit the establishment of the ability to vibrate?
Question
Is there a possibility for the Middle Self
to understandably depict the subtle perception?
Information reaches the conscious mind
Most subtle perceptions are withheld through this process

manner, then ask friends to be your model. If that doesn't work, use photos or paintings of people for whom there are biographies. Yes, you read it right—you can also do aura and energy-field readings on the basis of such material! But always look at the biographies only after you have done enough readings and interpretations. Don't let yourself be discouraged right away by information in the life descriptions that seems contradictory at first glance. A number of biographies are sometimes necessary (and you can find stacks of them in any public library) to get a rounded picture of a person. And if you really do make a mistake at some point, then remember that Rome wasn't built in a day either. Learn to do it better next time by carefully analyzing your mistakes.

I would like to make some further comments about how information is processed through the Inner Child. Each of us constantly absorbs subtle information of all kinds through the level of the Inner Child. This information has its own quality—like smelling, tasting, hearing, seeing, and touching. But we haven't had any training for thousands of years in dealing directly with these very personal subtle sensations. Although we can perceive them, our Inner Child hasn't agreed upon a "classification table" with the Middle Self, the conscious portion of the personality, to which it could refer when imparting perceptions from this region in order to help the conscious mind understand its messages. So the Middle Self must help us in order to once again learn how to interpret the subtle sensations. Just like the linguists, once they have become familiar on site with the language, also prepare a dictionary for foreign languages in which anyone can read, for example, what "yes" or "dog" means in Kisuaheli, you must now work together with your Inner Child (which we could say is on site) in order to prepare a translation table for the subtle area of perception. In this way you can define certain blocks as black or gray, typical chakra energies as red or blue, and naturally also subdivide a person's energy system into the various defined levels.

All of these aids in understanding are naturally just symbols. When a Bushman sees an airplane, he probably describes it to a fellow clan member as a very large, shiny metallic bird that doesn't even move its wings when it flies, strangely enough. As long as the other person understands what the first one has said, then everything is fine. The communication works! Accordingly, the chakras don't have any specific color. But the system of the spectral colors is particularly well-suited for being able to comprehend and interpret the processes and qualities of the energetic events within them. The chakras themselves don't really exist as we generally understand them to exist. The system of chakras, the meridians, etc., is an approximation in order to be able to deal with the processes on the subtle levels. This is why there are different systems for describing and approaching the human energy system all over the world. And these also work. They are all maps and descriptions from various perspectives. As long as they can be put to practical use, they are correct and it's superfluous to fight about which of the systems is best. The more extensive and finely elaborated a description of subtle relationships is, the better we can work with it. Once you have understood this situation and no longer believe that your root chakra is actually red, then you have the freedom to be creative in dealing with the subtle energies.

The trusting work with your Inner Child (to which the same guidelines naturally apply as for the other descriptions) is extremely important for your possibilities of exploring etheric levels. Open up to it and you will make things possible for yourself that you hadn't even dared to dream of up to now.

With the following illustration, you can take a graphic look at the process of how the Inner Child treats and prepares subtle perceptions for the Middle Self. It's useful for you to understand these occurrences. Then you can more easily translate your own ideas into practical terms.

Perhaps this all appears boring to you now, but do yourself the favor and take it seriously. Although you are still dependent on black/white readings at the moment, except if you have already snooped around in the next chapters, these can still be very profound and comprehensive. Don't pounce on the exercises for reading the aura in color too soon but first work extensively through the exercises described in this chapter. At school you didn't start right away with integral calculus either but with 1 x 1. Particularly to ensure clean work in the subtle region, it's important to take one step after the other and not proceed too hastily.

In the next chapter we will then come to the highest art of non-color aura-reading, perhaps even of reading the aura at all: reading and interpreting chakras with the ancient Chinese Book of Changes, the I Ching.

Chapter 6

The Chakra Oracle—Reading and Interpreting Energy Fields with the I Ching

As we conclude the non-color methods of reading the aura, I would like to present you with a very special goody: reading chakras with the I Ching! This ancient Chinese oracle system and book of wisdom, which is at least 5,000 years old, has been ascribed to the legendary saint Fu Hsi in its original version. About 4,000 years ago, the wise King Wen and his son, the Duke of Chou, wrote an extensive commentary on the rough draft. And about 2,500 years ago, the great philosopher Confucius penned a further comprehensive accompanying text for it. All of China's significant teachers of life and philosophers, such as Lao Tse, Mo Ti, or Dschou Hi, were inspired by the I Ching. Its advice has been used by musicians in composing and playing, by writers in authoring books, by doctors in the treatment of patients and preventive health care, and by warriors for tactics, strategy, and the development of highly effective martial arts. Even in modern times, this book has hasn't gone out of fashion. Mao Tse-Tung, for example, asked the I Ching whenever he needed advice.

There is hardly an area of Chinese culture and civilization that hasn't been and isn't profoundly influenced by the I Ching.

The Book of Changes—as the I Ching is also called—has been a loyal friend and wise teacher to me for well over twelve years because it describes the world as involved in constantly flowing change. Perhaps it seems odd to you that I talk this way about a book, but when you have gathered some experiences with its oracles, its loving, sometimes quite original and direct manner of giving you advice for your development will certainly tend to impress you as a living being instead of a collection of printed pages.

However, I don't want to go into the customary oracle work with the I Ching in this chapter. During my involvement with this book and the philosophy upon which it is based, it has become clear to me that the I Ching basically describes the current overall state of the chakra system in its information, called hexagrams. Each hexagram is, as the name implies, made of these six lines placed on top of each other. The individual lines are either solid, describing a yang energy, or broken, which means a yin energy, or they are called changeable lines. This means that a line is still in the yang state, for example, but changes into the yin state (or vice versa).

I have checked this time and again for many years and, without exception, it's been confirmed that each of this six lines describes the energetic quality of a main chakra. This means that the first line (always from the bottom!) describes the quality of the root chakra, the second line the quality of the sexual chakra, the third line that of the solar plexus chakra, the fourth that of the heart chakra, the fifth that of the throat chakra, the last and sixth that of the forehead chakra. In case you are now asking what happened to the description of the seventh main energy center, the crown chakra—well, that's quite simple: it results from the combined state of the other six main chakras.

As described in Chapter 4, the crown chakra represents our divine consciousness, or the consciousness of unity. According to the degree in which I've found a unity of my body-mind-soul on the levels represented by the lower six chakras, the state of my seventh chakra will change. Whenever the I Ching shows one or more changeable lines in the information, the crown chakra will change as well. Sometimes this occurs in the direction of more divine consciousness, and sometimes in the direction of less. Unfortunately, I can't give you a comprehensive description of the many application possibilities and interesting background of this discovery here.

However, this isn't absolutely necessary in relation to the art and science of reading auras. You can get a great deal of use from this application of the I Ching if you carry out some basic exercises with it and spend some time on understanding the necessary theoretical backgrounds.

This chapter, the explanations of the main chakras in Chapter 4, and a good I Ching book (see bibliography) will serve as the basis for your own discoveries. In the following, I will show how you can read the chakras in the sense of the I Ching and how hexagrams derived in such a way can be interpreted as an overall picture according to the chakra theory. On the basis of the six hexagrams, we will work through some examples of interpretations together. Once you have carefully gone through all of this, it shouldn't be difficult for you to carry out simple interpretations of other hexagrams yourself.

Since, as extensively described in the last chapter, your Inner Child is the part of your personality responsible for energetic perceptions, the chakra readings related to the I Ching must be preceded by an agreement with it regarding what it should do and how it should impart its perceptions to you. One simple method of doing this is a fantasy journey into this area of your being. The following text should serve to guide you in it. It isn't important for you to use it word-for-word. Go ahead and adapt it to better fit you personally.

A Journey to Your Inner Child

Sit down or lay down in a relaxed way. Close your eyes. Sense your feet and legs. Now tense all the muscles in this area. Then let go again. Wait a few breaths. Now sense your lower abdomen and pelvic area. Then tense all the muscles there. Let go again. Wait a few breaths. Sense your chest, stomach, arm, and shoulder area. Now tense all the muscles there. Let go again, and wait a few breaths. Sense your throat and head area. Tense all the muscles there. Let go again. Wait a bit and then feel your way into your breathing rhythm.

Now say softly: "I would like to have contact with you, Inner Child—please respond!" When you have a distinct signal for the contact (an image, bodily feeling, sensation, etc.), ask for its cooperation in learning to read the chakras with the I Ching. Tell it to clearly respond when it feels you are demanding too much of it and would like a break. Promise that you will respect its needs and make sure that they are fulfilled as well as possible at the first opportunity. Then explain to it that you have the desire to perceive the six main chakras (root chakra, sexual chakra, solar plexus chakra, heart chakra, throat chakra, and forehead chakra) within yourself and in others by seeing the subtle energies. In doing this, you would like to see the yin state of an energy center as a broken line, the yang state as a solid line, the change of a yang to a yin line as a solid line with a small circle at the center, and the change of a yin to a yang line as a broken line with a small x in the space. Each line should be visible in the area of the chakra that is to be described. (Before the fantasy journey, look at the illustrations of people with the hexagram lines drawn on them so that your Inner Child can better understand how it should depict its perceptions.)

Thank your Inner Child once again for its cooperation and take leave of it.

Pay attention to the flow of your breath for a while, tense all the muscles in your body, take a few deep breaths, and then open your eyes.

The Interpretation of the Individual Hexagramm Lines

The following themes are represented by the individual lines (from the bottom to the top):

1. Hexagram line: Root chakra (survival/fight and flight/reproduction in the sense of preservation of the species/the fulfillment of fundamental needs/instincts)—"Earth" as the area of existence—This deals with human concerns closely linked to the material world.

2. Hexagram line: Sexual chakra (relationships/joy in life/meaning and fulfillment linked to material things/reproduction in the sense of joy in resonating along with the cosmic process of creation/the feeling of unity with the world/taking care of personal interest in the sense of "how can I experience the beautiful things that do me good?")—"Earth" as the area of existence—This deals with human concerns closely linked to the material world.

3. Hexagram line: Solar plexus chakra (use of power/manipulation of substances and energies when the respective person comes into contact with them in order to absorb things that are necessary in the most beneficial form and incorporate them into his own system and eliminate, restructure, or place the non-beneficial things in such a way that they cause as little damage as possible when they stay/setting limits/living individuality)—"Human being" as the area of existence—This deals with human concerns closely linked to the material world that affect existence as an individual (egocentricity, to not necessarily be understood in the negative sense).

4. Hexagram line: Heart chakra (accepting the substances and energies that the respective person meets with, without "if" and "but"/ socially acceptable actions and thoughts/love that isn't connected with sexual attraction)—"Human being" as the area of existence— This deals with universal ideals that cannot be materialized in reality without solid anchoring in the area of human concerns.

5. Hexagram line: Throat chakra (expression of personal energies in actions and consciousness, active shaping of the surrounding world. In contrast to the third hexagram line, this isn't concerned with acting when something enters the realm of one's own personality but active self-expression, the willful representation in the outer world/ communication/resonance of being)—"Heaven" as the area of existence—This deals with universal ideals that become an end in themselves without use for the rest of the world without solid anchoring in the area of human concerns (lines 1–3).

6. Hexagram line: Forehead chakra (empathy, recognizing and following one's own path/wisdom in dealing with oneself and others based on the knowledge of cosmic order and the conscious acceptance and lasting understanding of the laws of eternal change/understanding)—"Heaven" as the area of existence—This deals with universal ideas that cannot be realized when they aren't solidly anchored in the area of human concerns (lines 1–3).

Within this context, the expression "earth as area of existence" in the explanations of the hexagram lines 1 and 2 means that these two areas are absolutely necessary for existence in the material world. If a being isn't interested in its survival (line 1), then it won't be on the earth for very long. If no relationships (line 2) are permitted, there will be no experiences with the world and the species will die out because of lacking reproduction.

Within this contact, the expression "human being as the area of existence" in this explanation of hexagram lines 3 and 4 means that these two areas are absolutely necessary for human life. If a person isn't in the position of living his individuality and intelligence (3rd line), then he cannot make his own very personal contribution to shaping the Creation. He also cannot live in a community (4th line) if he doesn't have what is probably the strongest human survival talent, mutual support through loving acceptance of the others. The human being, who is quite a weak creature on his own, will therefore have difficulty in surviving under such circumstances.

Within this context, the expression "heaven as the area of existence" in the explanations of the hexagram lines 5 and 6 means that this area is absolutely necessary in order to bring the heavenly creative energies to the material level. This ability of self-expression (line 5) is a reflection of the divine ability to shape the world according to one's own image. A sense for recognizing and following one's own path in relation to the rest of the Creation (line 6) makes it possible for a person to shape his life in all of the five other areas so that it helps him and the surrounding world to further develop the Creation and therefore make a harmonious contribution to the realization of the divine plan on the material level.

Interpretation Examples of Six Hexagram Lines within the Context

When interpreting the individual lines, pay exact attention to including the correlation with the rest of the hexagram. Lines that should actually be seen as having an inappropriate energy for their place, such as a yin quality on the first line, can be totally "right" if their energies are meaningful within the scope of the overall hexagram. Perhaps this sounds a bit complicated at the moment, but it's quite simple in the practice since there are many good books on the I Ching in which you can look up the necessary information on the meaningful interpretation of a hexagram when reading chakras. In this respect, my comments in this chapter are just meant to give you some ideas as to the background of the hexagram interpretation and not replace a complete treatment of this topic, which would go beyond the scope of this book.

Well—and now we can start with the first practical exercise. Make yourself comfortable in your practice room, put a pad of paper and pencil next to you, close your eyes, and in your mind ask a question about your life. It shouldn't be a "yes/no" question, and it should also be unambiguous. This means you shouldn't ask about a number of different things at the same time. Here are some examples: "What is the basis for my relationship with (name of your intimate partner/

a parent/friend/relative/colleague, etc.)?" or "Why is it so hard for me to stop (for example, smoking)?" or "What's my mood like to-day?".

Then ask your Inner child to show you the state of your chakra system as a hexagram, meaning with lines corresponding to an energy quality for each chakra. Next, use your inner eye to look at the areas of the six main chakras and note the lines that you perceive at the individual energy centers, starting at the root chakra up to the third eye. Always go from bottom to top, like a tree grows.

Once you've written everything down, thank your Inner Child for its help and look up the interpretation of the hexagram in the I Ching book. When you have taken an extensive look at this, try to understand the meaning of the hexagram based on the energetic condition of the chakras, which is described by the individual lines. You can facilitate this work by reading through and understanding the six interpretation examples in the second half of this chapter.

At the beginning, everything is bound to seem strange and perhaps difficult to you, but if you "stay on the ball," reading the chakras with the I Ching will soon be fun and very simple for you. This is one of the most intensive methods for interpreting the energy system within its context that I know. Instead of being concerned with the state of the individual energy centers in an isolated way, you can use the Book of Changes to understand in relatively easy way why a chakra is in a certain energetic state right now and what consequences result from this in relation to the other chakras.

If, instead, you interpret the chakras individually when reading the aura, you may easily come up with the wrong overall interpretation. We could say that reading chakras with the I Ching is the high art of aura-reading. The more intensively you work and feel your way into this method, the more your interpretations will gain in quality and depth.

Just like you can read the condition of your chakras through a hexagram, you can also do this for other people. Simply add a chakra-reading with the I Ching at the end of the normal process of reading the various levels (see last chapter). It's best to only give your interpretations and advice to the client after you have become clear about the meaning of the hexagram that you have observed in him or her.

At the beginning, only ask about things that relate to you! This type of questioning the I Ching is by no means a substitute for the oracle methods with a random generator like coins, yarrow sticks, and other similar approaches since your ideas in relation to the question can very much have an influence on what you see. With much practice and the development of a neutral attitude in the I Ching work, the two methods increasingly approach each other in terms of their objective quality. However, for difficult questions I always recommend working with coins or similar methods of questioning.

However, subjective information is not only adequate for our purposes but also even desirable. Once you have learned to work with the I Ching as a method of reading the chakras, then you can use this in a quick and confidant way to determine in a reading how a person relates at the core of his personality to a certain issue. The disclosure of this attitude is a great help in passing on advice that the other person can also accept and translate into action. Or, it can also help in getting a new perspective for the interpretation when an energy state is difficult to interpret. Combined with the other perceptions, a meaning will result. When reading energy fields and auras, we basically always work with subjective attitudes since a human being's difficulties just happen to be subjective.

Interpretation Examples of Six Hexagram Lines in Relation to the Chakras

No. 1—Creative

In this hexagram, all of the lines are yang. This means that every chakra has energies that express themselves, have an influence, and want to manifest themselves. In accordance with this, a person in this state tends to have a desire for action, has ideas, and also has the necessary strength and ability to turn them into action. This can become a problem if he takes on too much in the long run and oversees his own limitations or those of his surrounding world in his state of creative frenzy. Sensitive souls in his environment may feel themselves pushed up against the wall just because of the power of his energy development. Family and friends are often neglected during such phases because the entire attention is concentrated on the creative process. On the other hand, these are the phases in the

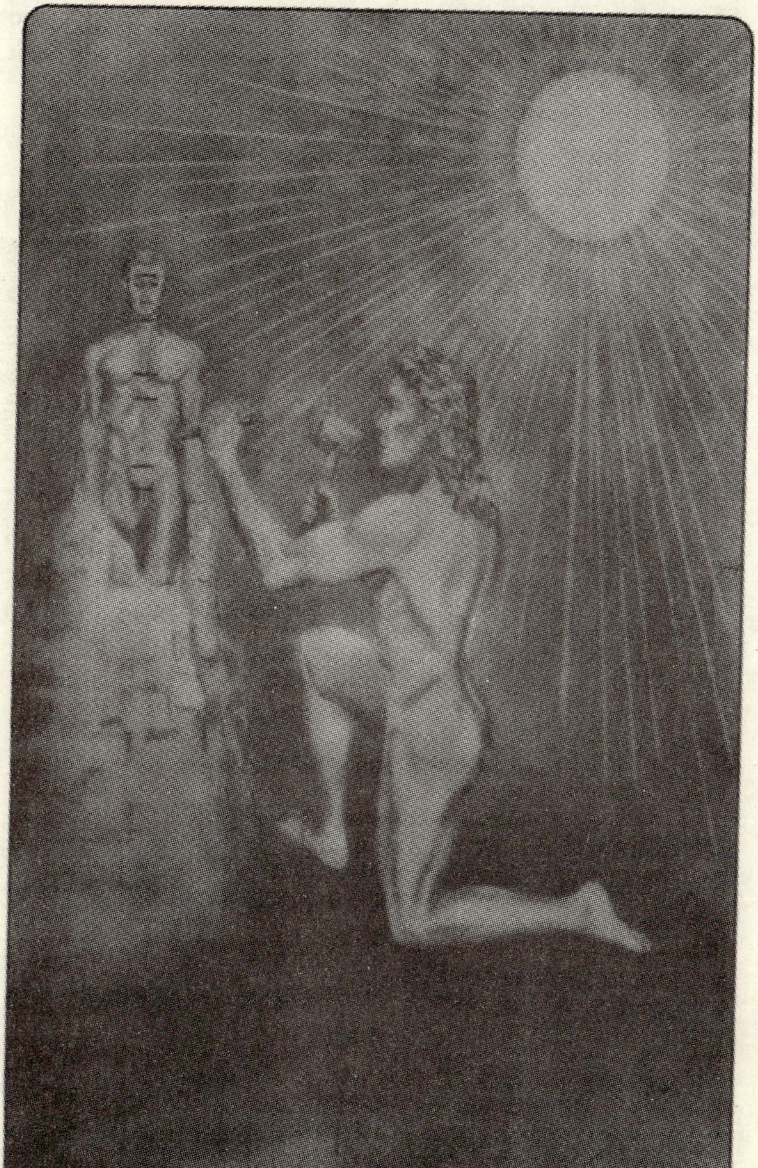

I Ching Hexagram 1 "Creative"

life of a human being that bring the "path of heaven" to earth and thereby the realization of ideas that serve one's own development and that of human society.

No. 2—Receptive

In this hexagram, all the lines are yin, meaning that all the chakras are receptive. This describes a state that is ideally suited for complementing the first hexagram, which is the creative force and creativity, in that it is willing to accept this energy. If a yang energy meets a yin energy, all the preconditions are fulfilled for this idea taking form. If the architect of a building project is yang, then the bricklayer who puts the stones on top of each other according to his instructions is yin. By the way, Hexagram No. 2 is the ideal energetic state for a woman who wants to have a child. In this process as well, the energies of an individual who isn't yet incarnated wants to take form on the material level here. A person who wants to live the mystic ideal of "Thy will be done, O Lord!" must have such a constellation in the area of his main chakras. This also applies to someone who wants to learn something, but his teacher should tend to have a chakra constellation as in Hexagram No. 1.

No. 11—Peace (Harmony)

While both of the first two symbols are quite easy to understand, things will get a bit more difficult now. This hexagram has yang lines in the lower three places and yin lines in the upper three. The instinct of self-preservation is therefore strong; there is an active striving for the realization of joy in life and relationships, as well as the ability to manipulate the energies and substances coming to an individual so that they don't harm but have a constructive effect.

The heart chakra with its yin energy is accepting and tolerant, causing no danger for the overall system since its necessary supplement in terms of setting limits against the absorption of influences that are too strong or harmful, the third chakra, is yang. The self-expression chakra, the state of which is described by the fifth line from below, is also yin and therefore creates no danger of the lower chakras' strong yang energies being used to attempt to imprint one's own individuality on others.

The exertion of power beyond the necessity of self-preservation, depicted by the third chakra, also represents no danger for contacts.

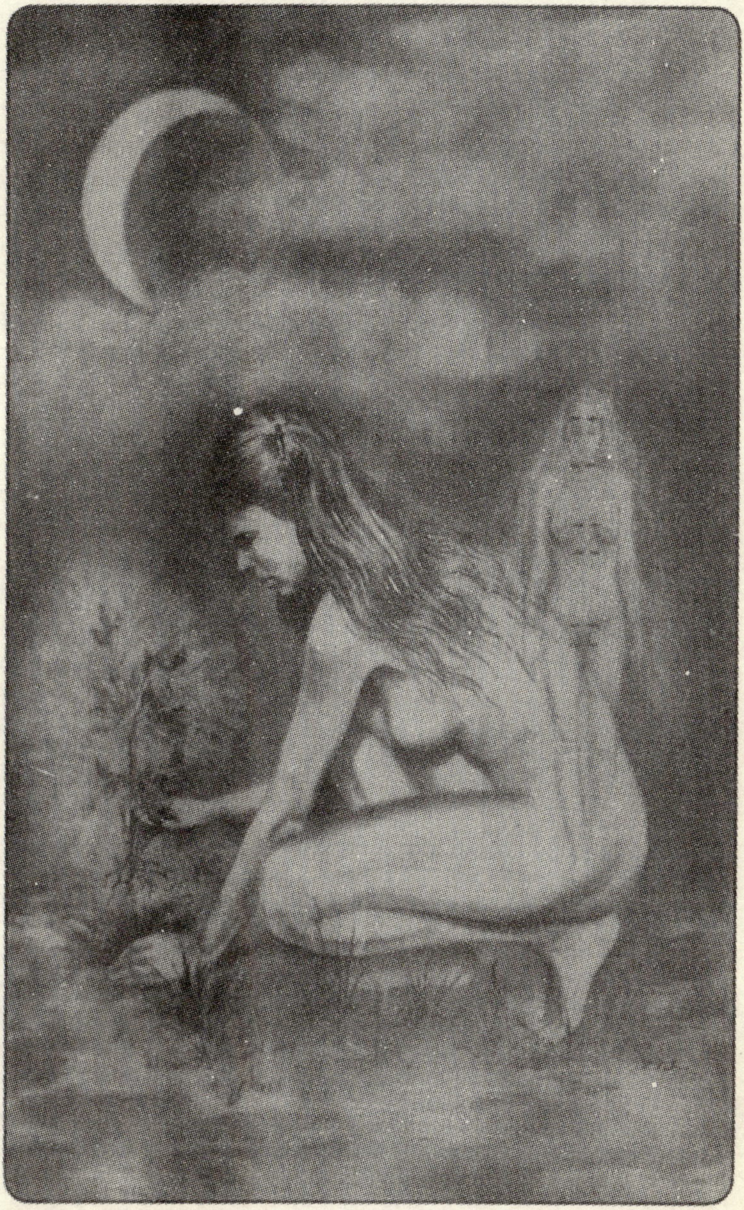

I Ching Hexagram 2 "Receptive"

Since the self-expression chakra is yin, there is even an increased perceptive ability of other people's self-expression. This openness for the self-representation of others is often helpful in taking the string out of critical situations in which a person can outwardly adapt for a certain period of time to the influences of others who are very intent upon self-representation, without this individual losing himself in the process. This is because his three lower chakras are so strong because of their yang power that he can remain true to himself on the inside. An image for this is the blade of grass that bends beneath the power of the wind yet isn't blown away because of its solid rooting in the earth and its elasticity. When the wind stops blowing, it simply springs up again and assumes its original position.

Because of its yin quality, the third eye (sixth chakra) is receptive to guidance by the cosmic vibrations. These give the person the ability to follow his path in life, no matter how complicated the situation, which is important and right for him within the overall context of the Creation. At the same time, the strong yang chakras in the lower region provide the power and the grounding for us to take the proper path. Accordingly, no obstacles are put in the way of a person growing and thriving.

The sole risk is that he will think this wonderful state is a matter of course. He may then no longer be concerned with perfecting his being or may let his roots get weak because of the ease and lose his sense of reality. He may also become intolerant and accuse others of being at fault for their own misery if they don't do everything right like he does (immodesty in a state of affluence).

You will often find such a harmonious constellation in a likeable, successful businessman who, to your surprise, also has spiritual interests. This hexagram also symbolizes the time of pregnancy, during which this structure of the chakras is necessary in order to let a new human being grow and take form. (Compare this hexagram with No. 2, which symbolizes the ideal state of receptivity for the chakras.)

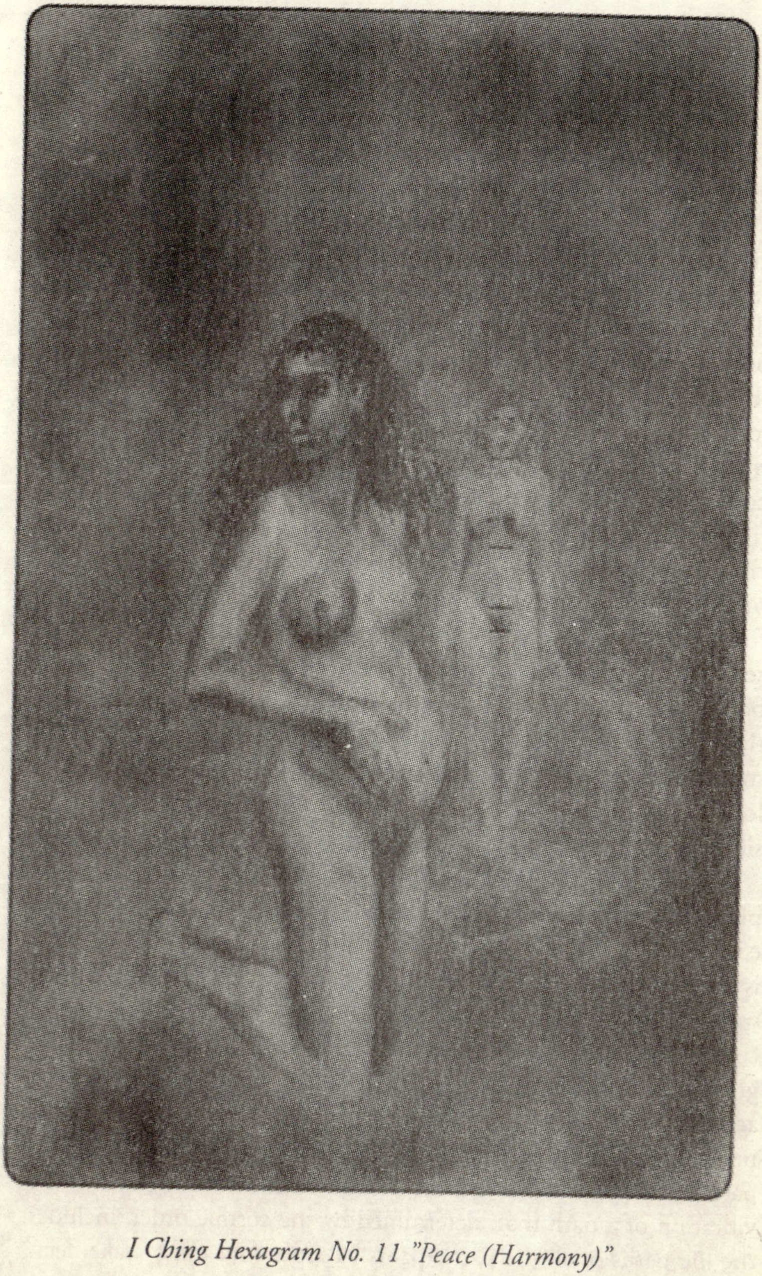

I Ching Hexagram No. 11 "Peace (Harmony)"

No. 61—Inner Truth

This hexagram expresses a state of deep perception. The root chakra (first line) is yang and therefore strong enough to secure survival. The relationship chakra is also yang. This state lets the respective person have an active approach to relationships (with himself as well!). The solar plexus chakra is yin and at the moment all energies come through as they are to the inside of the body-mind-soul. In general, this can lead to difficulties, yet the benefits prevail in this hexagram. The lower two lines are strong enough in order to protect the vulnerable middle for a while, if this is necessary. In this case, the weak third line helps perceive the world and oneself for a time without glossing over things. That a person must refrain from manipulating and setting limits is an unavoidable precondition for coming into contact with the real truth. As soon as the third chakra carries out its normal activities, a person will only come into contact with the appropriately processed energies. The others, which cannot be reshaped, will be kept outside. In order for the contact with reality to also lead to a maturation of the personality (development of the heart chakra), the fourth chakra must be yin, meaning receptive. A perception of truth is possible through this center's tolerance. Without this quality, a situation is automatically created that produces confrontation. A peaceful way of looking at the truth and letting it have its effects is no longer possible.

The yang quality of the fifth chakra provides the ability to express the truths accepted in the heart region and let them become a component of self-expression. The yang quality of the sixth chakra is necessary in this constellation in order to not disrupt the contact with the comprehensive truth and the willingness to accept this by considering it from the perspective of the personal path. This hexagram deals with comprehensive truth. It can only be perceived and accepted from a superordinate perspective. This state of consciousness remains distant as long as a person orients himself on his own path. In order to achieve this state, he must attune himself to the vibration of a path that, determined by the cosmic order, includes the life paths of all the participants. People who must make decisions for others should be able to go into a state of inner truth so that they can consider the interests of all the people affected in the sense of the cosmic order.

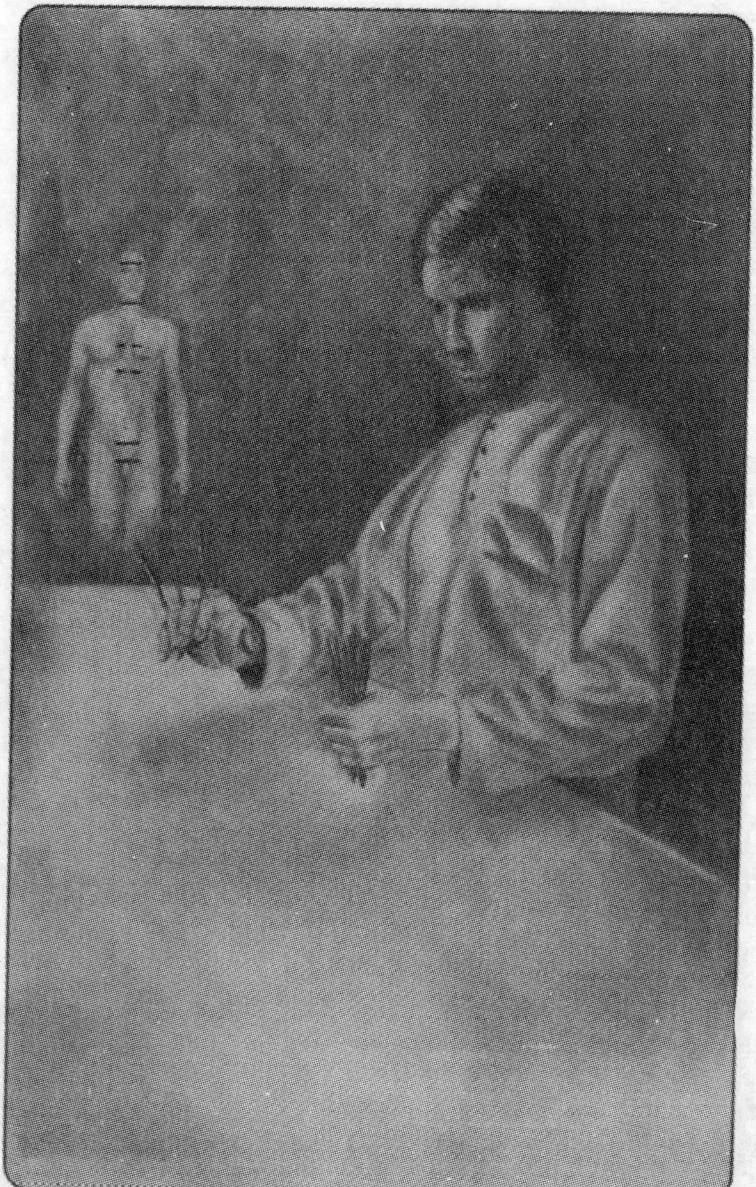

I Ching Hexagram No. 61 "Inner Truth"

No. 6—Conflict

This hexagram describes the state of the main chakras during a conflict. The first line is yin, and in accordance with this, the ability to actively secure survival by fighting or fleeing is not very pronounced. "Strange," is what you may now be thinking, " but this is about a confrontation?!". That's right, but a conflict usually occurs when someone is very vulnerable (open to attack, not adequately able to fight or flee).

The line of the relationship chakra is yang. So someone wants to actively enter into a relationship. But at the same time, he is more intensively looking after his own interests than wanting to open up to the other person.

The power chakra is yin, and therefore not in the position of keeping inharmonious influences outside or reshaping them so that they can be integrated harmoniously (vulnerability, not being able to put up with anything).

The heart chakra is yang and the abilities of tolerance and love aren't very pronounced. Since the throat chakra is also yang, the respective person will still have the urge to actively express his inharmonious condition caused by the constellation of the lower chakras and thereby attempt to influence his surrounding world. The others will feel disturbed by this and attempt to set limits. And now the conflict is already under way.

The sixth chakra with its function of guidance is also yang and therefore not open for the vibrations of the universe, upon which the "quarrelsome person" can orient himself in order to get out of his inharmonious mood and once again live in harmony with his surrounding world.

No. 52—Keeping Still (Meditation)

This hexagram is a symbol for the state of meditation. Every type of meditation! As you can see, the first line is yin. The root chakra with its basically active qualities of fleeing and fighting therefore tends to be passive. Instead of actively endeavoring to survive, an individual is depicted in a state of being protected here. The self-preservation instinct, as an important component of the ego, must be pacifying for successful meditation so that it's possible for the person meditating to simply look at his inner life with its sometimes threatening images without making any valuations.

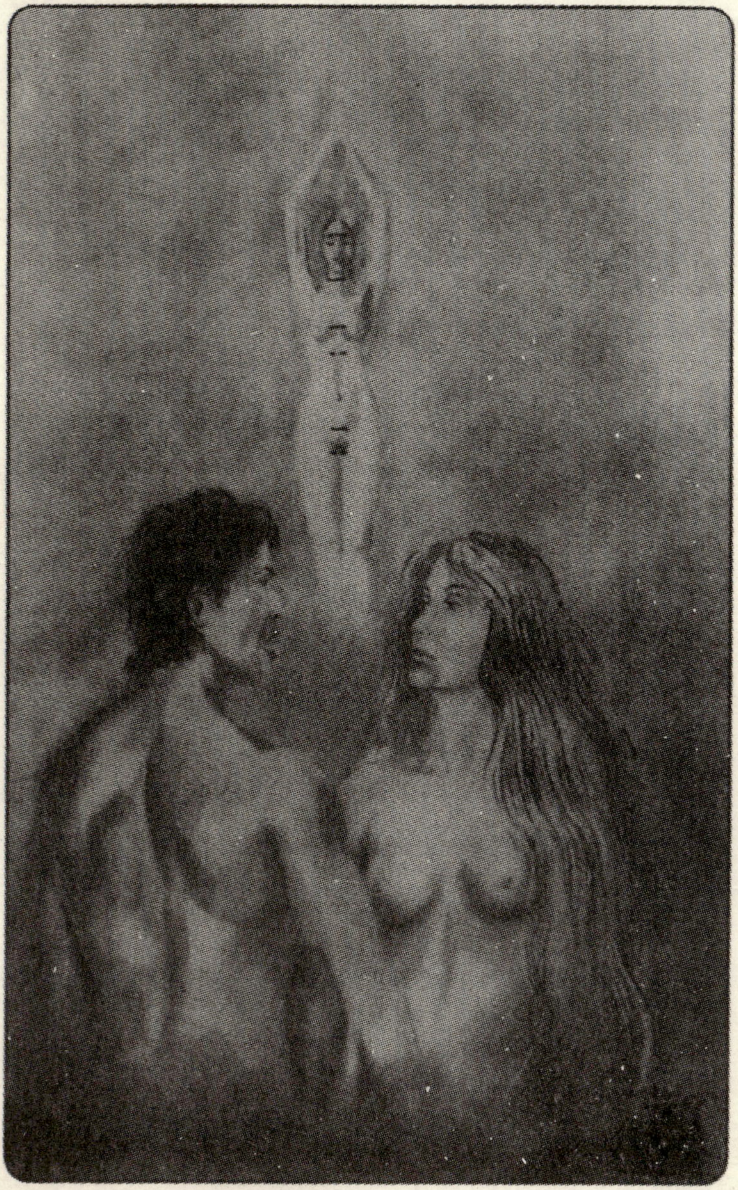

I Ching Hexagram No. 6 "Conflict"

Fleeing from this means once again somehow banishing these unconscious portions out of the conscious mind. Fighting with it would mean wasting valuable energy in a conflict with oneself, thereby making impossible the process of loving acceptance of dreadful images, which is the main thing that meditation deals with.

The second chakra has a yin quality since the greatest possible self-perception is absolutely necessary for successful meditation. However, since the surrounding world with its many influences is also perceived by the second chakra, the third chakra must necessarily be yang. In this way, the images rising up from the unconscious mind can be harmoniously integrated into the whole of the body-mind-soul on the one hand, and on the other hand it can treat influences coming from the outside so that they don't disrupt the inner processes.

Because a strong solar plexus chakra is important for meaningful meditation, all spiritual traditions oriented toward practice place a great deal of value on its development. They emphasize that meditation should only be done with an empty stomach since this energy center will otherwise be almost fully occupied with digestion. There's a saying that "the well-fed have no use for books!" If the body is occupied with the utilization of food, then it has little digestive capacity free for mental impressions, for which the same center is responsible.

By way of contrast, the heart chakra is yin so that it's easier for the person meditating to lovingly accept the dark sides within himself that he recognizes during the practice. To the same extent, the center of self-expression is also yin since meditation is concerned with everything other than showmanship. This would only detract from the occupation with one's own inner life.

The sixth chakra has a yang quality. Why should it? Well, a person who meditates generally has the desire to be attuned to his path in some way. He hasn't yet achieved this, since otherwise he wouldn't have to practice. In the ideal case, the yang energy in this chakra is aroused by a mantra (holy word), selected for the respective person by an experienced teacher and given to him to practice with, a breathing method, a visualization, or the like. This gives the practitioner special stimulation so that he will become increasingly good at perceiving his own path.

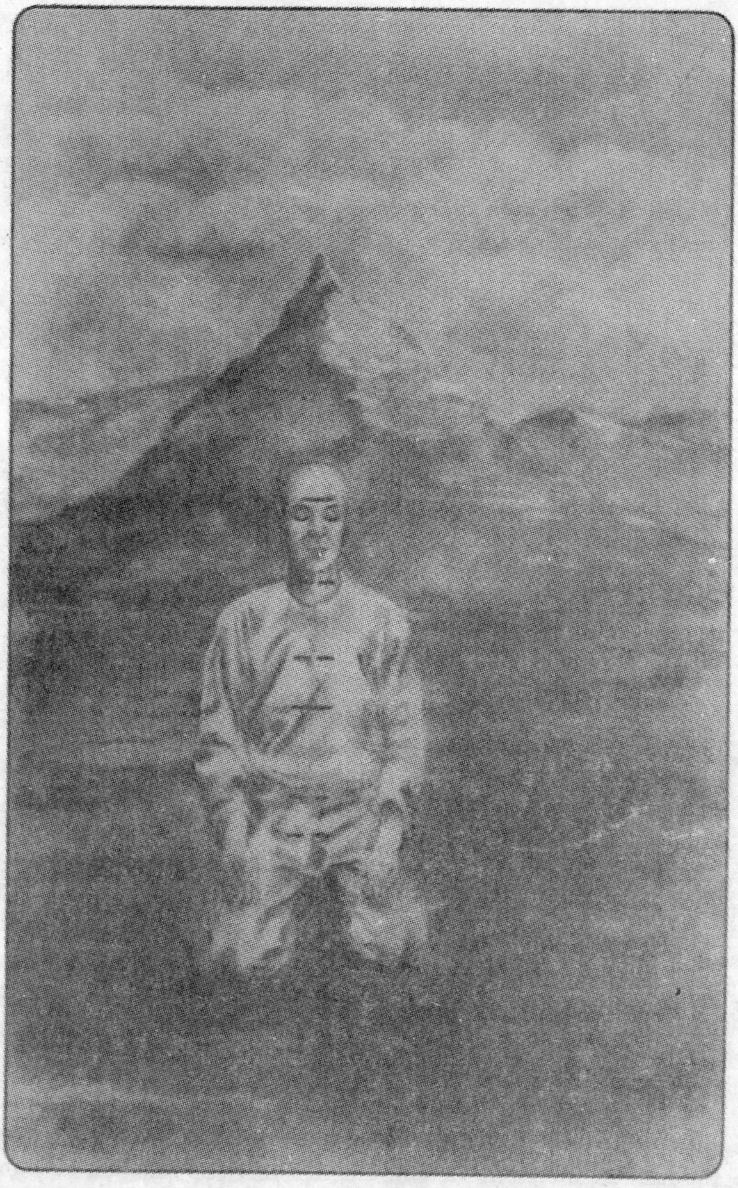

I Ching Hexagram No. 52 "Meditation"

If this energy isn't in the third eye, or if it is expressed in a way inappropriate for the practitioner at the moment, meditation won't function. The quality of the yang energy must also be adapted to the student's progressing developmental process time and again until the student has learned to adequately attune himself. This is why the Eastern meditation tradition places so much value on the practitioner being accompanied by a meditation master.

An Overview of Yin and Yang Qualities

Yin: the feminine; the north; cold; in the original meaning: the side of the mountain facing away from the sun; the moon; the inside; the cloud-covered sky; dark; the hull; spatial expansion; the material; performing; reacting; being treated; feeling; sensing; nourishing; resting; conditional; tangible; phlegmatic; melancholy; taking flight.

Yang: the masculine; the sun; warm; in the original meaning: the side of the mountain facing the sunshine; light; the core; the outside; the course of time; energy; idea; acting; creative; unconditional; intangible; sanguine; choleric; thinking; achieving; fighting.

Simple Meditations with the I Ching

At the conclusion of this chapter, I would like to describe one further method: doing a healing meditation with the I Ching hexagrams.

First consider in which area of your life you would like to grow. Then ask the I Ching with coins or yarrow sticks—as described in the relevant literature—for a hexagram that can help you in your development in this area. With this way of questioning the Book of Changes, you turn directly to your Higher Self and can receive information that is sound for you in the holistic sense. Make a large drawing of the hexagram found in this way on a piece of paper. Now you can start the actual exercise.

Relax, close your eyes, and make contact with your Inner Child. Ask it to help you attune the energetic state of your six main chakras to the energy of the hexagram. Then simply direct your attention to your chakras and watch how they slowly adapt to the desired quality. Look at them in their totality for about five minutes. Then thank your Inner Child, take a few deep breaths, briefly tense all your muscles at once, and open your eyes.

Repeat this exercise as often as you like. Stop doing it if you feel an aversion to it. If this aversion persists, let the I Ching give you a new hexagram. Even though this exercise is quite simple, it can set a great deal in motion!

Chapter 7

Exercises for Color Perception of Subtle Energies

So, now we can finally start with the color perception of subtle energies. I'm sure you've been waiting for this.

Before you start with the actual "training," request from your Inner Child in the manner that you've been accustomed to that it cooperate with you. In this way, the part of your body-mind-soul that has direct access to the subtle levels is prepared for the coming journey of discovery and learning.

The following color-perception exercises should help you increasingly differentiate your ability of perceiving the subtle world and make practical use of this ability. So that you can correctly interpret your observations, you should first become familiar with the theory of the energy system, the interpretation of the colors as described in the next chapter, and the systematic structure of an aura-reading as described in Chapter 10. You can naturally also do this parallel to the exercises. You can always look things up at the corresponding place in the book.

Color-Perception Exercise 1

Put yourself in the state of inner vision as described in the chapter on reading the aura in black/white. Ask your Inner Child to also let you perceive the colors and look at the various levels of your aura. Also compare this with the descriptions of the aura in Chapter 4 and the information in Chapter 9 about how to do a reading and interpret the aura and its fields. Make detailed(!) notes about each level of your perceptions.

In the beginning exercises, an extensive set of colored felt pens served me well. The drawings with the colored pens save you a complicated description of the colors that you've seen.

Color-Perception Exercise 2

When you have precisely described the individual areas of your aura and made sketches of them, then take your perceptions to the area of your main chakras. Use the felt pens to draw each of them extensively with all the details, with each of the chakras on separate standard-size pieces of paper. Although these exercises may take a while, and you shouldn't do them all in one session because of the necessary effort at the start, they do make a great contribution toward developing your abilities of differentiated color perception in the subtle area. Moreover, it's great to draw your chakras in all their rich colors. These exercises have always been a journey of self-discovery for me as well and I really enjoy expressing myself artistically in this manner.

By the way, don't worry if you aren't skilled at drawing. Just simply do it—you will be surprised at the wonderful results. If you practice with a group (see the epilog), then it's very worthwhile to discuss your chakra pictures and aura sketches together in detail, helping each other mutually in interpreting them. You should also make some brief written descriptions of the aura and the chakra system in order to practice recognizing correlations and fluently formulating what you've observed. This is very important for when you do readings for other people later. You will probably have a bit of difficulty at first in finding all the appropriate words. Then work with the descriptions and pictorial comparisons. It's important to find a language suitable for expressing your observations in the subtle area so that you can also think about them more easily and talk to others about them.

Color-Perception Exercise 3

Use your inner vision to observe your rings of muscle armor and pay attention to whether the energy qualities are stuck there. If so, look at where they are stuck. You will perceive the corresponding colors and can deduce from them what chakra energies are blocked in which areas of your body.

Color-Perception Exercise 4

Use your inner vision to observe specific secondary chakras, one after the other, and make note of what color they take on, dependent on your mood. You can then change your mood using different kinds of music, fragrance oils, incense, chakra meditations (for example, with the *CHAKRA MEDITATION* CD/cassette by Baginski/ Sharamon, Inner Worlds Music, which are particularly well-suited for this purpose), or the preceding fantasy journeys. Do these exercises on all the secondary chakras described in this book and make precise notes about the readings.

Pay attention as to whether certain energies have a hard time appearing in the observed secondary chakras, or perhaps don't appear at all, and how clear the colors are in the process. These exercises will not only make the work more routine, but also will give you an improved intuition about the moods and feelings behind certain colors in the secondary chakras, as well as their source (relation to main chakras) because you have experienced these yourself. It is very important for the development of all areas of subtle perception to have extensive experiences yourself. You can more easily perceive things in others, understand their deeper meaning, and interpret the observations in practical terms within their context when you have experienced all this and felt it yourself.

Color-Perception Exercise 5

Use your inner vision to observe the subtle function of your main organs and meridians, as extensively described in Chapter 4. Look at the color qualities and interpret them within the context of your observations on the levels of the main chakras, secondary chakras, and the aura.

When you have had enough experience with observing and interpreting your energy system, you can go on to doing readings of historical individuals for whom there are biographies available. You can also train with friends or in a work group of like-minded people. However, at the beginning you should really just practice on yourself. Otherwise, you won't have a true understanding in your mind and belly of the processes in the energy system.

Chapter 8

The Meaning of the Colors in Subtle Perception

The meaning of the colors when reading the aura is very significant. Both the color itself, as well as its mixture with other colors, its luminosity, clarity, or shading with black or white reveals important information about the energy qualities that these symbols are based on. So that you can better understand the description of the individual colors within this context, I would like to give you some basic information about the theory of colors as an introduction.

The Rainbow Colors, Black and White

All colors of the rainbow (spectral colors) are created from white light, the united totality of the individual colors, such as they are broken within a drop of rain and thereby separated into components. The rainbow symbolizes the state of unity, loving togetherness. In it, we can observe that all colors have their meaning and are harmoniously connected with the others. If one color is left out or too strongly included in this color mixture, then the result will no longer be white since the equilibrium has been disturbed. In accordance with this, all colors are equally important. None is "better" or "worse" than the others. This situation is very interesting in relation to the interpretation of the main chakras' colors. If the color of one or more main chakras is too strong or too weak, then the seventh chakra, the crown chakra, which reflects a person's state of loving self-acceptance, cannot develop into radiant white.

The colors are created in that all the other partial vibrations of the white light are absorbed by a surface and only the color vibrations visible to our eyes are reflected. A material that appears to be white accordingly reflects all vibrations—it doesn't let anything get into it. In keeping with this, a clearly distinct white in the energy system can express a strong need for protection (I don't want to be hurt/touched!) or it can be a sign of arrogance (Leave me alone with your nonsense! The others aren't important! and so forth), or it may be consciously applied by spiritual teachers and therapists in order to be a perfect mirror for the others. Through this quality, the student/client is confronted with all of his aspects—even his suppressed aspects that he usually tries to hide so well from himself and others.

As an energy quality, white can also show up in the aura when the respective person has completely accepted himself and sends out a strongly loving vibration on all levels. The developed crown chakra then outshines all the other vibrations and also colors the aura in the process. I call this an "active" white to differentiate it from the "passive" white that has the effect of letting nothing get close to it. However, this active state is very rare and you probably won't be able to observe it in one of your clients. If you see it at all, it would probably be in a person from whom you are seeking advice. So white can hardly be interpreted in the isolate state.

If you notice this energy while reading an aura, always pay exact attention to the various different functions of the related parts of the energy system in order to come to a conclusive interpretation. According to my experience, white can usually be observed in people who protect themselves and in those who can't accept anything, who don't want to be confronted with reality. White therefore has a strong connection to the solar plexus chakra (fears, power, and manipulation).

Keyword for White: I Don't Want to Have Anything!

The opposite of white is black. In the narrower sense of the word, this quality isn't a color either. We perceive black when a substance absorbs all the partial vibrations of light without any differentiation. In a certain sense, black is also the color of love, the unconditional willingness to accept, and thereby closely connected with the energies of the heart chakra. The surrounding colors attain a stronger luminosity through black; it increases their individual expression because, resulting from its quality of unconditional acceptance, it creates an environment whose radiance doesn't compete with the other energies. Black also stores energies. If you wear clothing of this color during the summer, you will get much hotter than if you wear, for example, a bright white wardrobe that keeps all the energies away from you.

Black in an energy system shows, among other things, that a person needs energy. Very exhausted, weakened people frequently show this coloration. You will also find black in the aura when people have so blocked the flow of their life forces that they depend on sucking the vital energy of others. People intensely involved with black magic in some form also tend to show black. This is why black is often seen as the color of magic, which it certainly isn't. In the practice of black magic, the realization of personal wishes stands in the foreground. Since these are seldom identical with the wishes of the universe, it doesn't provide them with any support either. So the magician must work with individual energy, which usually can't be regenerated all that quickly and must also be mobilized to a substantial degree since the person is now also swimming against the universal life flow. These substantial energy problems show up as imbalances in the area of the first chakra and strong blocks in the area of the sixth chakra. The conscious or unconscious sucking of other people's vital forces (psycho-vampirism) is then seen as an apparently easy solution. However, this solution only works for a limited time because the solar plexus chakra is constantly overloaded as a result.

To make a long story short: this is why the color black is associated magic and in no case should you take it on sight unseen. Just like when dealing with the color white, first take a precise look at the overall energy system before you come up with an interpretation. As the color of the willingness to accept, black can also always be observed in attentive students and generally in people within whom a strong interest for some sort of perception has been awakened. Black is also the learning color. And finally: blocks often appear black since the body sucks energy at these points in order to hold onto it. You will rarely see a pure black in blocks since this is usually a strongly shaded complementary color to the energy that's intended to be held. The body has good reasons for selecting what should flow and what should be congested.

Keyword for Black: Give Me Energy!

An extensive understanding of the many aspects of black and white is very important in order to be able to grasp the meaning of the various light and dark tones of the colors when reading auras and comprehending the fundamental mechanism of energy direction.

Black and white complement each other in a meaningful way in order to enable the vital energies to flow and keep them in motion. A symbol for this is the yin/yang monad, which comes from China. Don't make the mistake of simply interpreting these colors to mean "good" and "bad"!

The Six Main Colors

When discussing the following six colors, I refer to the color table printed on the back side of the book cover. It's important for you to have an optical impression of the colors that I mean. If you look at the squares, you will discover that the colors have a somewhat unusual effect. This is no surprise since they are ideal colors.

Red contains neither black nor white, nor yellow, nor blue. The same applies to both of the other basic colors, which are printed without mixing in any other colors. The mixed colors are made of 50% each of the two colors. So orange is half red and half yellow, green is half yellow and half blue, and violet is half red and half blue. Otherwise, there is nothing else in them, which is why they look somewhat strange. In real life, you will hardly ever see these tones during a reading. They are just ideal colors. But now that you know how these colors look when they are truly pure, you can more easily identify and interpret shadings of all types. These shades occur in the chakras, for example, when an energy center is overlapped by another or is closely linked with it at the moment because they have a task to fulfill together. In the first case, the one chakra is shaded but not the other one, which is influencing it. In the second case, both colors are somewhat enriched by the respective color of the other chakra.

If a chakra is shaded with black, this tends to mean a willingness to accept energies. In order to make your interpretation, you must relate this chakra to your observations within the rest of the energy system.

If a chakra is shaded with white, you can assume that energy is kept out for some reason here. You can discover why by relating this to your further observations.

The Three Primary Colors Red—Yellow—Blue (the Yang Energies)

These colors represent the basis for all other color mixtures. Although they can be shaded darker through black and lighter through white, their energy quality can only truly be changed by mixing them with other colors. In this respect, they are an expression of the primal energies that produce all the others to a certain degree. In accordance with this, they are also yang and associated with the yang chakras: RED—root chakra; YELLOW—solar plexus chakra; BLUE—self-expression chakra.

The Meaning of the Color Red

Red is probably the first name of a color that was used at the very beginning. This is no wonder since red symbolizes the will to incarnate in the material world. If it's missing in central areas of the energy system or is only faintly present, the result is a weakened will to exist. Only in the rarest cases will this be a direct death wish, but usually does mean a weakening of the primary vital forces from which all possible imbalances could naturally grow. A dominance of red indicates there is a fight for survival in the foreground of how a person lives.

When it shows up in partial areas with a great radiant power, this can indicate inflammations that are latent or already manifested on the physical level, which can be attributed to conflicts that haven't been lived out. Allergies often draw attention to themselves through a red gleam in the affected areas, shaded with the colors that symbolize the qualities triggering the allergy. An energy that harmoniously complements this quality is the green of the heart chakra. Green directs excessive red energies into appropriate, growth-promoting paths and stimulates the formation of red energies when they are too weak. This serves to also explain the connection of the heart chakra with the immune system, which is basically associated with the root chakra but must be activated through the heart center.

In the balanced relationship with the other colors, red indicates vitality, dynamism, a good sense of reality, the ability to be motivated, a general abundance of energy, and a life shaped according to both cosmic and individual factors.

Also include my interpretation of the root chakra when dealing with this color.

In organic terms, red has a connection to the MESODERM, a type of body tissue that grows from one of the three so-called germ layers (middle germ layer) after a human being has been conceived. Later, the skeleton, connective tissue, muscles, urogenital tract, spleen, blood vessels, heart, and blood cells are created from this germ layer.

The astrological signs of Leo and Aries are also associated with this color.

KEYWORD: Energy of the will to exist.

The Meaning of the Color Yellow

Yellow is the most radiant of the primary colors. It is the color of the midday sun's light. The vibrations of yellow symbolize resolution extending to the point of decomposition. This is why the "digestive chakra," the third chakra, is related to yellow. It is also the color of the thinker and philosopher, the analyst, and the wise ruler who translates the laws of heaven into reality on earth. The first emperor of Chinese history, who simultaneously was a great teacher of the people and a type of saint, was called the "Yellow" Emperor (Huang Ti). In China, this color was generally associated with the emperors. In Central Europe, yellow has greatly conflicting meanings. During the Third Reich, people seen as outcasts, like the Jews, prostitutes, and women with illegitimate children were made to wear a yellow mark.

What has produced such contradictory interpretations? In my opinion, this resulted from the difficulty of dealing meaningfully with the energies symbolized by the color yellow. In order to fully develop the wisdom and virtually superhuman qualities of this vibration, a person must experience all the heights and depths of life, understand their meaning, and have lovingly accepted this. Only then will power no longer be used on the basis of fear, greed, and aversion, but according to the divine will. True wisdom and love can't be learned from books or dry discussions. Only an experience that has been worked through and integrated without prejudice can develop these qualities. Christ's way of the Cross and Hesse's novel *SIDDHARTHA* very vividly show the development of the color yellow's radiant power. Although many people consciously or unconsciously search for it, they get stranded on the darker sides of life instead of accepting this experience as a purification.

A "sage to be" who is going through a necessary "gutter experience" for his development in order to continue on to other, "nicer" areas of life with deeper insights and a greater ability to love is hardly different from someone who gets stuck in a difficult life situation and doesn't know how to get out of it, and maybe has even given up the search for a way. Few people are aware of this correlation. Yet, the deeper knowledge of its special characteristics is expressed in the different valuations of the color yellow.

Because the perfect radiant power of yellow is a necessary precondition for developing the ability to love in the fourth chakra (green), which is therefore dependent upon this, the solar plexus has a primary color associated with it and the heart center has a mixed color. This correlation results in profound consequences. Think these through carefully and sense them within yourself because it's very worthwhile to do so. I don't want to take this work away from you since comprehending certain correlations on your own is vitally significant for your personal development.

When interpreting yellow during a reading, pay special attention to its clarity and radiant power. If the yellow tone is somehow shaded, the possible wisdom and clear ability to judge may be obstructed by the energies that are mixed in with the yellow. This is particularly interesting with respect to people who say that they live based on their feelings but in reality tend to have their intellect impeded by firmly held and falsely directed energies, which can be seen through intense color mixtures in the yellow areas. But this intellect still attempts to determine what happens in their lives.

Pure violet can harmonize excessive yellow—for example, constant brooding with results that aren't turned into action—by bringing the analytic energy in contact with the ability to perceive and thereby triggering the motivation to act.

Also refer to my statements on the third chakra when interpreting this color.

In organic terms, through the ECTODERM type of tissue, which develops from the so-called outer germ layer, yellow is connected with the surface tissue (like skin), the sensory organs, the brain, and the nervous system.

The astrological signs of Gemini and Scorpio are related to yellow.

KEYWORD: Analytical energy.

The Meaning of the Color Blue

Blue is the most spiritual of the three primary colors. It is the color of material expression of the universal life energy, which can be clearly seen in water that is charged with it, as an example. In a reading, you can use the blue tones in the energy system to see which individual varieties of the universal life energy would like to express themselves or cannot express themselves. A dark shade tends to mean an obstruction of the expression, a light shade tends to express the energy but is somehow "disguised." When someone expresses a feeling of envy (yellow shade) in the form of apparently objective criticism, you can see a light shade of blue with dark yellow tinges. For the deeper interpretation, always look at the energy centers that have similar colors. A radiant, pure blue can only be seen in the self-expression of a person who has learned to completely accept himself. By the way, blue light has a calming effect and can be harmonizing for inflammations and irritations. Contact with the symbol for the universal life energy that penetrates everything reduces conflicts. Communication (energy exchange) and understanding for other people is promoted in this way.

Pure orange can harmonize excessive blue by directing self-expression based on a craving for recognition for its own sake back into healthier paths of self-expression for experiencing the self, therefore leading to a more meaningful and fair exchange of energy.

For the interpretation of blue, include my explanations on the fifth chakra.

In organic terms, blue is connected through the ENTODERM type of tissue (inner germ layer) with the surface tissue ("lining") of the digestive tract (functions: protection, exchange of substances, reception of stimuli), the parenchyma (function-bearing tissue), the tonsils, thyroid gland, parathyroid gland, thymus gland, liver, pancreas, the lining tissue of the urinary bladder, the ureter, and some areas of the inner ear.

Cancer and Taurus are the corresponding astrological signs.

KEYWORD: Energy of expression.

The Three Primary Mixed Colors Orange—Green—Violet (the Yin Energies)

These colors result from the mixture of two primary colors respectively. They accordingly symbolize the unification of various qualities and can therefore be classified as yin. This results in their association with the yin chakras: ORANGE—sexual chakra; GREEN—heart chakra; VIOLET—third eye. Mixed colors symbolize the realization of the ideas of the primary colors in the material world.

The Meaning of the Color Orange

Orange is a mixed color of red and yellow. It materializes the will for existence and for analyzing manifestations in the material world through openness for relationships, and by enjoying and desiring them, which makes all types of relationships more stable and solid. Experiences are made possible through orange. Pure blue can stabilize excessive orange and thereby contribute to not getting lost in the experiences, which would mean living through them without using them for the benefit of one's own development and seeing their only purpose as "having a good time." Orange can always be helpful when a person has lost the ability to enjoy life. People who have lost touch with reality, who believe they can only live in higher realms, can regain their sense of reality through orange.

KEYWORD: Experiential energy.

Associated energy center: Second chakra.

The Meaning of the Color Green

Green is a mixed color consisting of yellow and blue. It materializes the ability to analyze the manifestations of the material world under spiritual perspectives. If you understand the world in its course of events in a earthly/logical way, but don't comprehend the divine meaning behind all of it, you will ultimately(!) hate it and despair because of it. However, if you can combine the radiant pure yellow of the sun with the transcendent blue of the heavens, you will achieve a state that is generally known as enlightenment. This enlightenment always grows from the contact of the pure blue with another color. However, it is the "enlightenment of the heart," which is symbolized by a clear green, that perhaps has the most profound effects on life and particularly the way in which a person deals with experiences. It's no coincidence that green is the color of harmonious growth and of plants, whose active substance chlorophyll enables them to connect the energies of the sun with the components of the material world.

KEYWORD: Creative energy (If you are now wondering why this isn't the "energy of love": The Creation is love that has taken form. Think about this for a while and don't stop if the consequences of this thought shake up your concept of the world!) Excessive green can be harmonized through pure red. In concrete terms, this can mean the restoration of a healthy will for self-assertion after a phase of self-sacrifice for the sake of others.

Associated energy center: Fourth chakra.

The Meaning of the Color Violet

Violet is a mixed color composed of red and blue. It represents the unification of the unconditional will for existence on the material level with the orientation of this enormous power toward the laws of universal life energy. In other words, this is a spiritualization of the will to exist. In a reading, pure violet always shows a far-reaching harmonization process. The respective person is therefore involved in shaping his entire life or partial areas of it so that it corresponds with his personal destiny in harmony with the requirements of the universe. Excessive violet can be harmonized by a pure yellow. If you are now trying to figure out why violet is inharmonious in large amounts: Someone who does everything right is no longer capable of learning to love and grow through the exertions with the challenges that must be mastered. Hexagram No. 63 in the I Ching describes this situation very well. It isn't the purpose of our earthly existence to be perfect but to have experiences and learn to love from the consequences of accepting our imperfection. A person who consistently does everything right will therefore stand in the way of both his own development and that of others since everything is connected with everything else.

KEYWORD: Energy of perception.

Associated energy center: Sixth chakra.

Chapter 9

Aura Reading in Practical Terms

Now that you have become thoroughly familiar with the theory and practice of reading auras and energy fields, and have already had enough experience to do the first sessions for others, I would like to give you some tips and advice about the structure and course of an aura reading. Similar to other counseling activities, there are modes of behavior and organizational methods that can make the work much easier for you.

Appropriate Conditions for an Aura Reading

Since the energy field of a human being interacts with the energies and situations of the surrounding world, you shouldn't do intensive readings during a lunar or solar eclipse. Also refrain from doing them when your client is very stressed or dominated by strong feelings. You should also be well-balanced and not subject to time pressure. In case of doubt, it's better to postpone a session than to give false readings and interpretations on important topics.

In no case should you do an intensive reading for someone whose life themes are closely linked with your own (partner, relatives, friends) since you will then automatically be biased. The other person will also unconsciously make certain changes within his energy system associated with your relationship and the mutual themes. If another person's themes cause you to have strong emotional outbursts, then postpone the session and first clarify your problems for yourself. The more biased you are in approaching a reading, the less effective it will be.

The Time Frame

Plan about 1 1/2 to 2 hours time for the first session. It's important that the person, who must open up to you intensely during the course of the reading to benefit from it, has enough time to warm up to you. Offer a cup of tea and first talk about general topics so that the two of you can get to know each other. Even if your client insists on receiving information immediately, give yourself enough time. The calmness that you now allow yourself will pay for itself ten times over in terms of the reading's quality.

Establish a time frame when making the appointment and don't get involved in long, undisciplined discussions. Some people will try to convince you that their interpretation of the reading is correct and not yours so that they can continue to live in the protection of self-delusion. But they have come with the intention of bringing a bit more light into their life, and they should receive this opportunity. If you limit the sessions in terms of time, such discussions won't even arise and the interpretation won't be "disimproved." In the following sessions, I have had the experience that about one hour is completely adequate.

Don't agree to do any telephone consultations. Direct contact is particularly important at the beginning.

The Room

The room in which you do the aura readings should be quiet. If it's within your apartment or house, then you should hang up a sign during the consultation with the words: "Please don't disturb—except for the end of the world!" A little bit(!) of incense or a fragrance lamp with sandalwood can relax the atmosphere. But don't use any other aromas without informing yourself extensively in advance about their effects. Be certain that they will be beneficial for the planned session as well. Many people sometimes react quite extremely to patchouli or lavender, for example. Don't play any music since the energy system may strongly interact with it. Turn down the telephone. In no case should you answer it during the session! The same applies to the doorbell. Constant distractions interrupt the process of the reading and stop the two of you from building a trusting relationship with each other.

There shouldn't be any transformer boxes in the room, and the house shouldn't be located directly under high-tension power lines.

The Structure of the Reading

You have now learned a great deal about the human energy system. Because of this, you might even be somewhat afraid of not comprehending everything and interpreting it properly within the context. This concern is totally justified. You can do a very extensive and basically correct reading, yet still not come to a suitable result if you lose yourself in the details. For this reason, I've sketched the course of the initial reading and a follow-up reading for you. Once you feel secure, you will certainly find your own variations of these procedures. And this is how it should be as well. Up until this point, you can orient yourself toward my concept, which has been well-proved in the practice.

The Course of the Initial Reading

First ask whether your client is currently involved in medical treatment, any type of psychotherapy, or is being treated with homeopathy, flower essences, or the like so that you don't become insecure because of possible symptoms of healing reactions during the reading or go off on the wrong track. When these reactions are far-reaching, they can become conspicuous through quite a bit of chaos in the aura.

Then ask the client to remove watches, rings, and jewelry and put them in a place at least two meters away from him. Tell him not to cross his arms or legs, and that he should let his arms hang down beside the body. Relax and direct your attention to your inner vision. First determine what color predominates within him on the level directly related to the present. If this is a mixed color, determine what colors it's made of, which color dominates it, whether the color is shaded with white or black or clear within itself, and whether it is intense or pale. Then determine what color is least represented within the client on this level. Afterwards, carry out the same observations on the medium-term energy level and, in conclusion, on the long-term level. Are these colors pretty much in harmony with each other, do they complement each other, or are they inharmonious together? Are the medium-term and long-term developmental needs taken into consideration in the current approach to life or not?

On the basis of these simple observations, which I summarize under the term COLOR CHECK, you will have gained some basic perceptions about the current state of your client. During the rest of the reading, you can build on these. Then look at the various fields of the aura. Do they easily transition into each other? Are no colors gathered on the transition points? Are the fields free of excessive correlating energies? Can you determine a slight streaming from the top of the head to the hands and feet? Are no intensely distinct images in the fields? Are the colors clear and transparent, and do the emotional body and the mental body overlap none of the other fields? If all of this is true, then it's quite likely that everything is in order. If you notice anything conspicuous, note it on a copy of the form (energram record) that has been copied to at least twice its size, which you will find in the appendix. I call this second part of the reading the AURA CHECK.

Now look at the chakras one to six. You usually don't need to take the crown chakra into special consideration in most cases since its state results from all the others. Do all the chakras appear to have their ideal color, are they symmetrical, and generally round? Do they refrain from overlapping the neighboring chakras, and do they all have about the same size? Also check to see whether their connection to the inner energy system (on the spinal column) is blocked and that they aren't lopsided. You can best recognize this by looking from the side. In the main chakras, a lopsided position quickly leads to blocks because this obstructs communication with the inner energy system and impedes the flow of energy within the chakra. A lopsided position means that a chakra isn't oriented vertically from the body surface in its natural opening direction.

Sometimes you will also find a divided chakra, but this is a very rare phenomenon. However, you should know about it because of the consequences. A divided chakra looks as if a large chakra has one or more offshoots with their own opening and/or connection with the inner energy system. Only very severe traumas or long-lasting intensive oppressed conditions lead to such constellations, which are always accompanied by difficult mental and/or physical states of imbalance. Remember to advise this person to go to a good healing practitioner or doctor of homeopathy for a consultation.

If you find something conspicuous when looking at the chakras, make a note of it and draw the important structures as sketches on the form. Then take another closer look at the yin/yang chakras on the shoulders. To what extent are they developed? Are there differences in their radiant power and orientation? What is their coloring like? Also keep a record of this. I call this part of the reading the CHAKRA CHECK.

Now you have enough information for a thorough reading. You can find the starting points in the conspicuous aspects and in the comparison of the COLOR CHECK with the AURA CHECK and the CHAKRA CHECK. The energram record will also help you in structuring your observations. Now ask your Inner Child to show you the chakra that is crucially important at the moment (this significance isn't objective but based on the unconscious preferences of the respective person) for the organization of your client's life, as well as the one he neglects most extensively. Although you can usually clearly identify these chakras already during the COLOR CHECK and the CHAKRA CHECK, this approach will help you see things more clearly if you are uncertain.

Once you have comprehensively determined the momentary state of your client, look at the connections between the individual blocks so that you get an idea of their relationships with each other. If the overall picture isn't clear to you or if you want to go into more detail on special factors for some reason, take a look at the state of the individual secondary chakras, meridians, subtle organs, and bioenergetic armor rings. You shouldn't go any deeper during an initial reading.

Now it's more important to first quietly and tactfully explain what you have perceived. Don't overrun the person. Respect his vulnerable and weak spots. He didn't come to you to be hurt but to bring more light into his life with your help. Although self-perception is frequently painful, you can take care to bring the information across in such a way that the client doesn't yell "ouch!" right away and totally withdraw from you.

For these reasons, you also shouldn't give in to demands of immediately exploring karmic burdens, main learning lines, and the like during the first session.

Keep on hand a few addresses of doctors, healing practitioners, and psychotherapists who work in a holistic manner so you can send people with more severe problems to them. You can also make a list of books on topics that come up frequently to give to your clients.

You will find suggestions for this in the commented bibliography in the appendix.

The Course of a Follow-Up Reading

In a follow-up reading, first systematically approach the conspicuous aspects that you noted during the initial reading. Then you can go into your client's special questions and also start interpreting the individual chakra levels. When doing this, pay attention to the color quality, black/white coloration, intensified charging or lack of energy, and images. If you are unclear about the theme of one level, ask either your Inner Child for an appropriate picture or take another look at the overall constellation in order to get the information that you usually will find there. Chakra readings with the I Ching can give you very profound information for this purpose. Oracle work can also complete the picture, particularly when there are many influences involved. The pendulum (you can find pendulum tables in the appendix) can also be very useful. In order to test certain reactions, you can carry out the emotional-reaction test described in Chapter 4.

However, you shouldn't let yourself be enticed into doing too much because of the extent and great possibilities of your "tool kit." It's better to do less and be sure that your client understands all the information that you've given him, as well as also being able to accept it. If you make the mistake of wanting to show everything that you can do, the whole effort will degenerate to a bad show. It isn't necessary to read and interpret the energy system down to the last detail in order to give your client good advice for his growth. Try to develop an eye for what's essential.

In further follow-up readings, check the fundamental structure of the aura and the chakra system time and again, paying attention to the things that caught your attention during the last reading. This is very important since it may be that certain blocks within your client are dissolved in the course of time, new learning lines may be added, or new blocks constructed or lived out. You naturally must take these changes into consideration in your readings so that they remain up-to-date and don't take place under the false assumptions. The deeper you go with your interpretations, the more important the explanations on how to understand your statements will be for your client. Terms like blocks, karma, disrupted chakras, etc., can produce a lot of fears if they aren't explained. For critical topics, always be sure to make it clear to your client that difficulties can always be mastered and don't represent God-given punishments. These fatalistic convictions obstruct every type of healing process.

If your client desires a written draft of the reading, don't(!) give him your notes and the energram record but write a short essay in the following days based on them in which you describe all the important things in a clear and unmistakable way. On the one hand, this approach will protect you so that you are sure that things you didn't mean aren't interpreted into your catchwords; on the other hand, your client is much better served with a careful draft since everything that interests him will be understandable and in the proper context.

TAKE NOTE! It's often important to create a certain clarity in your client's energy system in order to directly answer concrete questions. There are so many important processes taking place in the body-mind-soul that it's only possible to answer these questions when everything irrelevant to this theme is faded out. It's quite easy to do this:

Ask your client to constantly think of his question or the topic that interests him while you do the reading. His energy system will then automatically become more active in the areas associated with this topic because energy will be collected here and be more passive in the areas not linked with it because the energy is flowing away from them. I call this method FOCUSING and use it quite frequently in the practice since it helps save a great deal of time and attention.

What You Should Absolutely Avoid During a Reading

- Never predict a person's death and don't make any dark insinuations!
- Never predict the future, except if you have a special talent for doing this, have had ample experience with it, know about the limitations and possibilities of prognoses, and are in the position of telling your client all of this in a very sensitive way!

- Don't make any diagnoses about organic or mental disorders if you aren't a doctor, healing practitioner with a certified license, or licensed psychotherapist! In the first place, it's irresponsible to diagnose diseases or make statements about their course if you don't really know what you're doing. In addition, you are committing a criminal offence if you do this.
- Don't tell any sort of "ghost stories" about possession, curses, black magic influences, or demons. Cases of this type are extremely rare. If you actually do encounter one, as long as you don't have any experience in this area and don't know how to deal with it, leave it alone for your own sake and that of your client. It's better to give him the address of someone who can handle such cases in a trustworthy and competent manner.
- In no case should you do readings for people who are seriously ill in the psychological sense.
- If you aren't healthy yourself, you shouldn't do any readings.
- You shouldn't do readings for people who just want to "test" you. It's best to keep such "curious" people away by asking a good price for a session.
- If you are in a hectic state or suffering from emotional stress, you shouldn't do any readings.
- You shouldn't do a reading for someone who you find totally unlikable.
- You shouldn't do a reading for someone in order to manipulate him in your interest or in the interest of someone else. Readings for the purpose of manipulation can lead to the partial or lasting loss of your abilities. Your Inner Child won't cooperate with this!
- Don't play the role of being mystical and secretive. Your clothing, the way you act, the way you talk, and the design of the room should be normal! Don't beat around the bush in order to show off, but get to the point.
- Don't work on photos of people that third parties bring you, except if the respective person has given you their written consent to do so.

Chapter 10

About Healing

You are now familiar with the many possibilities of perceiving and interpreting subtle phenomenon. In dealing with this exciting topic, you are certain to frequently have had the desire to help and support the restoration of harmonious states in a human being's energy system. There's nothing standing in the way of this if you are a doctor, healing practitioner, or certified psychotherapist. If you don't have a "license," then you are breaking the law if you make diagnoses or work therapeutically in the medical sense.

Today there are a great many self-help methods that are used by increasing numbers of people instead of chemical medications when less severe health disorders occur in the family or circle of friends. And you can naturally also become active within this scope to help your loved ones in a natural way. In order to give you a brief survey, which obviously can't be complete, I have listed some of the effective, easy, and safe methods that can also be applied by people who are not medical professionals. At the conclusion of the chapter, I've also included a few fundamental statements about healing and illness.

Aromatherapy

Healing with beautiful fragrances is becoming increasingly popular. It's no wonder since this method is simple, effective, and ... smells good! There is ample literature available in which you can find everything you need to know for using it in a meaningful way in the personal sphere. There aren't too many courses on this topic at the moment. If you do find one, get involved and expand your knowledge about it.

Biochemical Homeopathic Remedies

This is a simplified, but nonetheless very effective method of applying homeopathically prepared mineral salts in low and medium potencies. They are sold over the counter in pharmacies and are very economical to use. You can find literature about them in a public library with a good assortment of books and in the medical sections of bookstores. Biochemical homeopathic remedies are very well suited as first aid for home and travel. They include: Calcium fluoratum, Calcium phosphoricum, Calcium sulfuricum, Ferrum phosphoricum, Kalium chloratum, Kalium phosphoricum, Kalium sulfuricum, Magnesium phosphoricum, Natrium chloratum, Natrium phosphoricum, Natrium sulfuricum, and Silicea.

Bach Flowers

The English physician Dr. Bach intuitively developed this system of energetically effective essences, which are made of plants for the largest part. They are harmless, yet very effective, and available in pharmacies without prescription. There is abundant literature available on this topic. Energetic disorders of all types can be treated very well with Bach Flowers.

Gemstone Therapy

When gemstones are used in the proper manner, wonderful healing can be achieved. Gemstone therapy works on a purely subtle level and can therefore also be beneficially applied when the inharmonious states haven't yet manifest themselves physically but can be perceived in the energy system alone. If you want to become familiar with this method, you should visit a few seminars held by someone who has practical experience with it, in addition to reading about on the subject. There is a list of some related books in the bibliography.

Meditations

This is an excellent possibility of preventative health care and support of holistic therapies. However, meditations shouldn't just be taken from books. It's important to be accompanied by an experienced meditation teacher over a longer period of time, no matter what type of meditation you do, so that you don't lose touch with reality. Then the healing effects of meditation can actually develop.

There are a great many meditation techniques such as Zen, Transcendental Meditation (TM), Vipassana, Kundalini meditation, and heart meditation. Courses on these and the many other forms of meditation can frequently be found in any big city, with a vast number of books available on them.

One method that's easy for anyone to learn and effective in its application is Three-Rays Meditation, which is imparted by way of an energetic initiation. When this is practiced, the development of all the chakras is stimulated in a very gentle way. This form of meditation is also suitable for people who otherwise have difficulty with meditating.

Reiki

This is my "specialty" since I'm a Reiki Master. This method of transmitting the universal life energy is simple, accessible for anyone, and also very effective as a preventative method and path of personal development. A person who has been initiated into a Reiki degree by a traditionally trained Master can impart the non-polar, unity-promoting, relaxing energy of love as a channel and therefore facilitate the personal process of maturation, effectively activate the body's own powers of self-healing, and produce deep relaxation. In order to learn or practice Reiki, it's not necessary for you to have any particular lifestyle, do special physical or meditative exercises, have a specific system of belief, or follow a spiritual teacher. There is good literature on the topic, but it can't take the place of a Reiki initiation. You can learn Reiki from any Reiki Master trained for this purpose. Ads can be found in esoteric magazines and sometimes even in regional newspapers.

What Is Healing and How Does It Work?

For me, healing is the restoration of functions in the body-mind-soul that are natural, lively, and appropriate to the human being in their current state. Illness, which means an inharmonious state of the organism, is always(!) developmental stimulation for the respective person. We are in this world to have experiences and learn to love ourselves in our imperfection. So there is no life completely without health disorders because, among other things, we grow through them. But this doesn't mean that we are damned to suffer. If you become sensitive to the pending learning situation and open up to it in time, then health disorders will stay within the scope of a quickly passing light cold or the like.

So it's up to your decision-making power to determine how you want to have your life: If you get involved in the experiences and developments as they are contained within your life plan, things will go well for you because you don't need any heavy-handed "tips". But if you want to swim against the current and assert your will (which also includes excessive(!) use of positive thinking, affirmations, and other, ultimately magical methods), after the initial apparent success you will have a great many difficulties that will multiply the less you open up to yourself in the way YOU ARE. The same also applies to techniques of this type dressed up in such words as Jesus, God, angels, and the like. Just because love and God are mentioned, doesn't always mean that love and God are present.

We can basically differentiate between two paths of healing: On the one hand, health disorders can be treated symptomatically. This not only includes the therapy methods of orthodox medicine but all types of natural-healing systems, as well as the many variety of mental healing, as long as a maturation and development of the personality doesn't take place through the healing process. Evidence of this maturation is, among other things, a high degree of consciousness and assuming personal responsibility in shaping one's own life.

The other path always includes a process of developing the personality. Although this may be supported by the outside and sometimes only made possible through the appropriate measures, it must ultimately be actively and responsibly lived out by the respective person.

Through the first method, quick and impressive healing can often be achieved, which is why many people let themselves be fascinated by it. But this type of healing isn't lasting or may cause one health disorder to disappear but produce others that will become apparent sooner or later.

The second path always takes longer than the first, is more arduous, and requires the active participation of the afflicted person in the process of healing. But, as a result, this path effects a lasting and thorough harmonization that permits the respective person to become stronger, wiser, and more loving on the whole. After such an illness has been worked through, he will be better able to follow his own path and have learned a bit more about living on the basis of love.

A very good method for attuning yourself time and again with love and your own path in the context of the path of the universe is working with "I AM." This is how it goes: Take five to ten minutes of your time, make yourself comfortable in a quiet place, close your eyes, and think:

"I AM AS I AM BECAUSE GOD CREATED ME ACCORDING TO HIS PLAN. I AM AS I AM AND I AM BEAUTIFUL, FINE, AND LOVABLE JUST AS I AM. I AM AS I AM AND I RECEIVE EVERYTHING THAT I REALLY NEED FOR MYSELF WHEN I AM ATTENTIVE TO IT AND LOVINGLY PERMIT MYSELF TO ACCEPT IT. I AM AS I AM AND I AM A CHILD OF GOD. I AM AS I AM."

Once you have done this little exercise a few times, practice it while taking a train, a bus, or when you just happen to have a bit of time. You can also just do parts of it at one time. It's not meant to be affirmation work! So you shouldn't just suggest these statements to yourself and try to believe in them. They aren't intended to—and won't—exercise any formative power on the outside world. Instead, they direct your perception to the most neglected (because it's unrecognized) blessing in your life that is constantly there for you if you would just accept it. In order for it to have an effect, you only need to do it on a regular basis in order to focus your attention on this topic. Only by directing your attention will profound processes of development be initiated. You can also do a brief AURA CHECK and CHAKRA CHECK before and after this exercise. You will be astonished at the difference and the harmonious changes that result.

Please don't confuse this work with I AM exercises done in order to create certain situations like wealth or the like. These exercises are a part of the positive-thinking techniques, which also have their meaning and purpose in the world but fundamentally differ from the method mentioned above.

Healing is flowing along on the individual path with the stream of universal life energy. Illness, on the other hand, is swimming against the current, wanting to divert or dam it.

Medications or healing methods of any type can't take care of the pending learning experiences for you. They may facilitate them or make them possible in the first place—they can do this, but not more. You have to live life yourself!

Chapter 11

Epilog

I've very much enjoyed writing the *Aura Healing Book*. In the process, I've had a great many important new experiences myself, although I've long been involved with this topic and thought I would "just" write down my previous experiences when I started this book project. There were many things that I could only touch on because the space in one book is limited. Yet, I'm not unhappy about it. The book recommendations and suggestions in the previous chapter should show you enough possibilities of living and working your way into certain areas. I also think it's important to not have everything set in front of you by one person but to profit from the experiences and various perceptions of many. This also keeps us open for new perspectives and for learning in the general sense.

Your abilities to perceive subtle energies will virtually intensify and expand on their own if you train somewhat in the way that has been described here on the one hand and take them seriously and only use them in a respectful manner on the other hand. It would be misuse for you to show them off as a party gag, in order to make a good impression, or for "mass studies" because you simply can't believe that something like this works. The more you misuse them in such a way, the more you will lose contact with the subtle levels. Similar to the use of oracles, your subtle senses will develop on the basis of a serious attitude and atrophy if they are used for purposes that basically have no deeper meaning for anyone. Treat your abilities like a precious treasure—they're worth it!

Almost all the exercises in this book are structured in such a way that you can do them alone. However, I do find it very useful to start a little work group with a few nice people and learn together, gather experiences and talk about them. You can learn much more quickly in this way and have others who can give you tips and important feedback. In addition, you always have willing "test objects" and can also have your own perceptions checked by people who are familiar with this topic. If you don't know any people who would be interested in experiencing the adventure of rediscovering

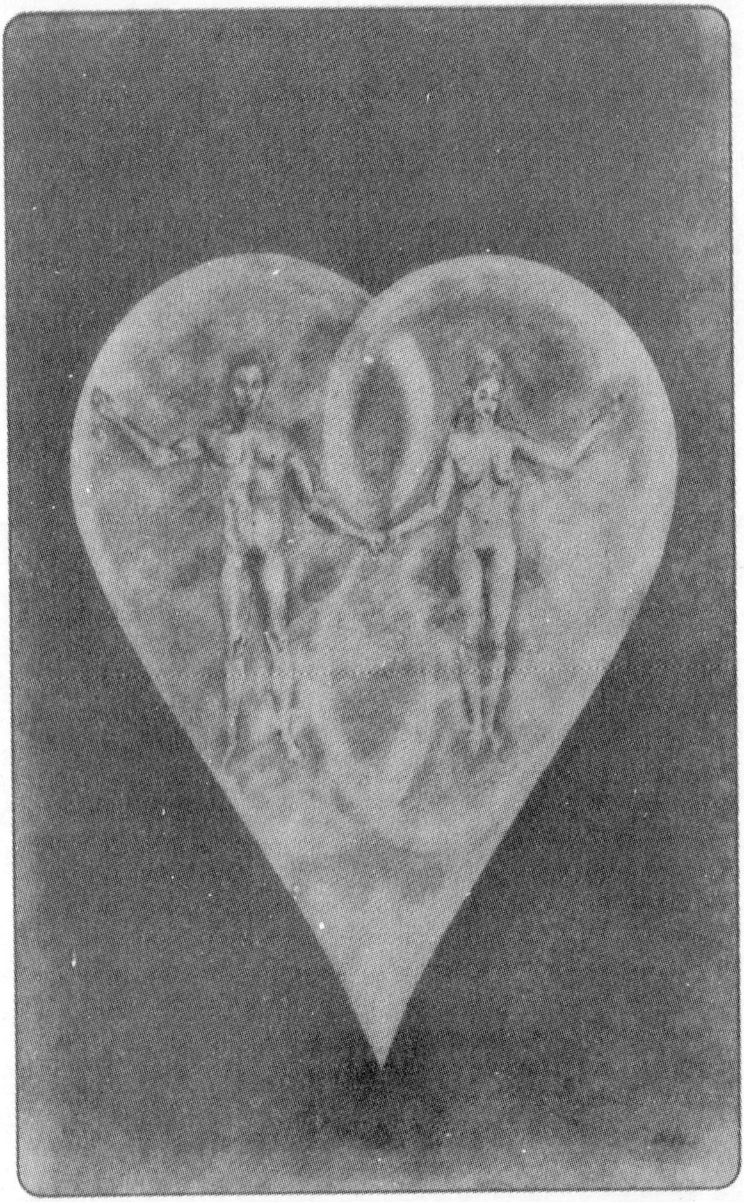

Learning to live in love

their subtle senses, then put a box-number ad in an esoteric magazine or a regional ad newspaper. The right people are sure to turn up.

One wish related to this book is to show you ways of shaping your life with more personal responsibility—to live it instead of having it lived. I have always had the experience that assuming the responsibility for one's own life is the most important developmental step in a human being's life at all. All other growth processes are only made possible in the first place by getting to know yourself and believe in yourself with everything that you are. In my opinion, loving self-realization in connection with the development of the universe is the meaning of our earthly existence. God is here and accessible for everyone, not just for "gurus" and "masters." And despite the undeniable usefulness of impulses that provoke thoughts and feelings provided by other people who share their experiences on the path with you, each of us can only find our own path to GOD alone.

I wish you love, light, joyful evolution, and that you can always accept God's loving blessing. It's always here for you.

Appendix I

The Direct Perception of Earth Rays and the Energetic Perception of Power Places

Although this isn't a direct part of reading auras, it's still a very exciting subject: the direct perception of earth rays and the emanations from places of power. Since an in-depth treatment would go beyond the scope of this book, I can only touch on this extensive topic. But, on the other hand, you've already received so many fundamentals in this book that it should be easy for you to do your own research. For this reason, I'm just going to give you some basic information.

Perception of Earth Rays

In the way with which you are already familiar, request that your Inner Child show you earth rays when you look at a room. Then switch over to your inner vision and pay attention to dark "whirlpools" in the room that turn to the right (waking zones, give energy) or left (take energy away). Then go to the place turning to the left with a friend and use the arm test (from kinesiology) to check whether the zone actually has a weakening effect. Then take him to a place turning to the right and carry out the test once again. This time, if you have seen things correctly, he should test stronger than before. Here's how to do the arm test:

Stand across from each other. One person lifts his stronger arm to the side until it's horizontal and places the other hand one hand's width beneath the neck on the thymus gland. The person doing the test then presses down the stretched arm by holding it at the wrist. Don't jerk when you press the arm down and don't do it too long in order not to tire the muscle. You just want to get an impression of its strength. After you know how strong your partner normally is, both of you should go to the place with the earth rays and repeat the test. But this time, the hand held on the thyroid gland before should now hang down next to the body and have its palm directed toward the earth.

Keep training this until you are sure of it. When doing so, change the location time and again so that you aren't influenced by bias.

The Perception of Emanations from Power Places

It's possible for you to look for conspicuous earth rays, as described above. But you can also observe the colors of a location using your inner vision in order to perceive its special quality, as well as identify particularly powerful places within this location in terms of their qualities and put everything into an overall context.

There are good books with photographs of power places from all over the world. In my experience, these are also fine for practicing.

Some power places have energy centers similar to the chakras in human beings, and it's also possible to discover an aura consisting of multiple levels at many of them.

Have fun trying this out!

Appendix II

Instructions for the Pendulum Tables

The pendulum tables are meant to help you find out the most effective treatment methods for the respective situation and, if you desire, carry out a somewhat more thorough search for causes. As I already explained in the main part of the book, such aids become dispensable with time, and this is good. But, until this happens, pendulum and oracle work can give you many good suggestions on how to approach the reading of auras. Since it's impossible to integrate all the alternatives in the tables, I have included some standard tables (tables 1 to 14) that have proved useful in the practice, as well as some additional tables without any entries on them. You can label these according to your own ideas and thereby create possibilities for analysis that are tailored to your own needs. You will find at least one field for "Errors" on all the labelled tables. This is important. Your pendulum will swing there when the table doesn't seem to have any appropriate statements or you can't receive any meaningful results with the pendulum for other reasons at the moment.

You can get a more detailed explanation of the obstacle with Pendulum Table 2 "Error Table." When you want to work on a matter that is very important to you, you should ask the pendulum time and again if the result is correct. In case of doubt, ask someone else who knows how to work with the pendulum and isn't emotionally connected with the question for advice. Supplementary oracle work with the I Ching, the Tarot, or runes is also very recommendable in this case in order to exclude errors as much as possible.

If you've never seriously worked with the pendulum or have little experience with it, you can take part in a good seminar, read a bit more about the subject (also see commented bibliography), and practice the simple exercises for a while before you work on important issues with it since the whole thing could otherwise really go wrong.

Pendulum Table 1

Cause of the Disorder

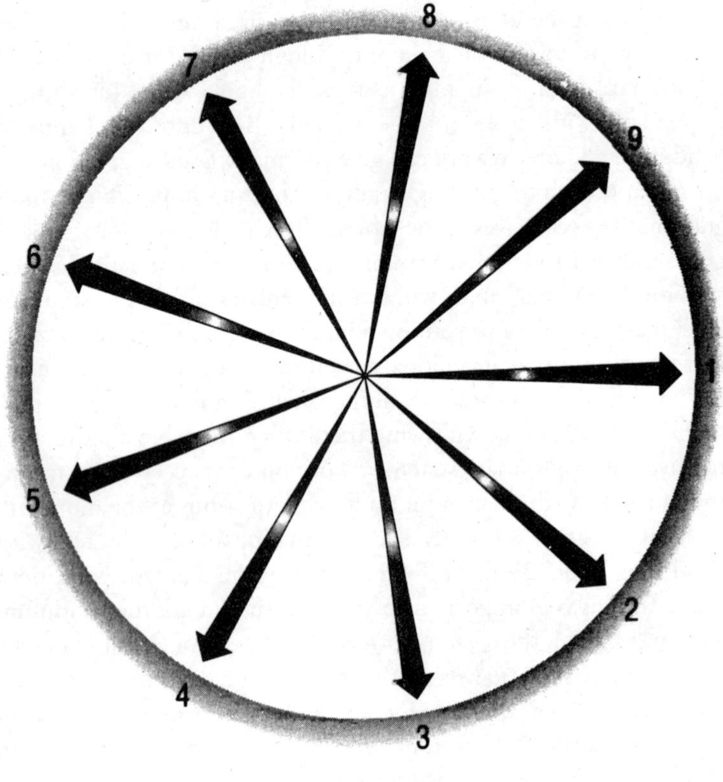

1. Error
2. Aura fields
3. Main chakras
4. Secondary chakras
5. Main meridians
6. Error
7. Energy meridians
8. Muscle armor rings
9. Organic

Pendulum Table 2

Error Table

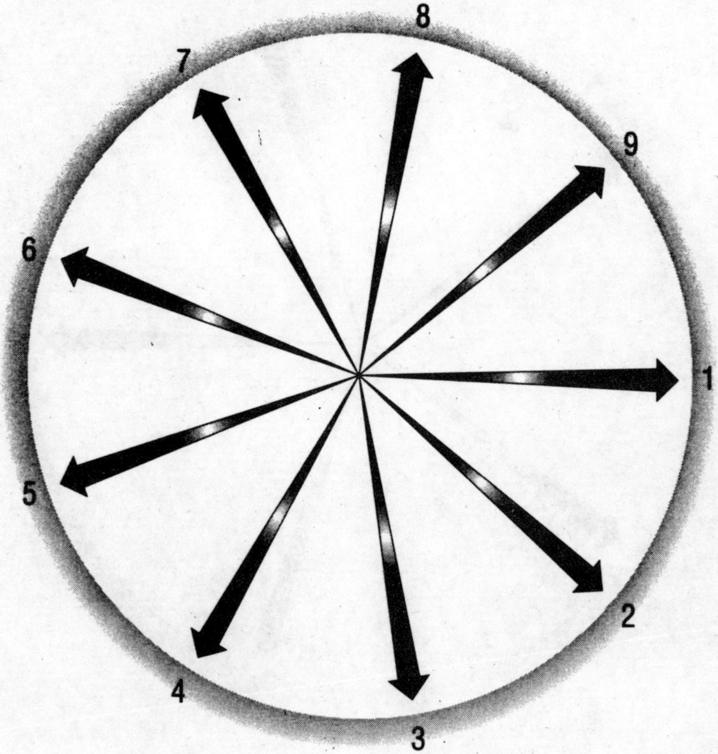

1. *You shouldn't work on this problem*
2. *Inharmonious place*
3. *Biased*
4. *Answer not on table*
5. *Too tired*
6. *You shouldn't work on this problem*
7. *Too rushed*
8. *Exceeds current ability to perceive*
9. *Own*

Pendulum Table 3

Aura Fields

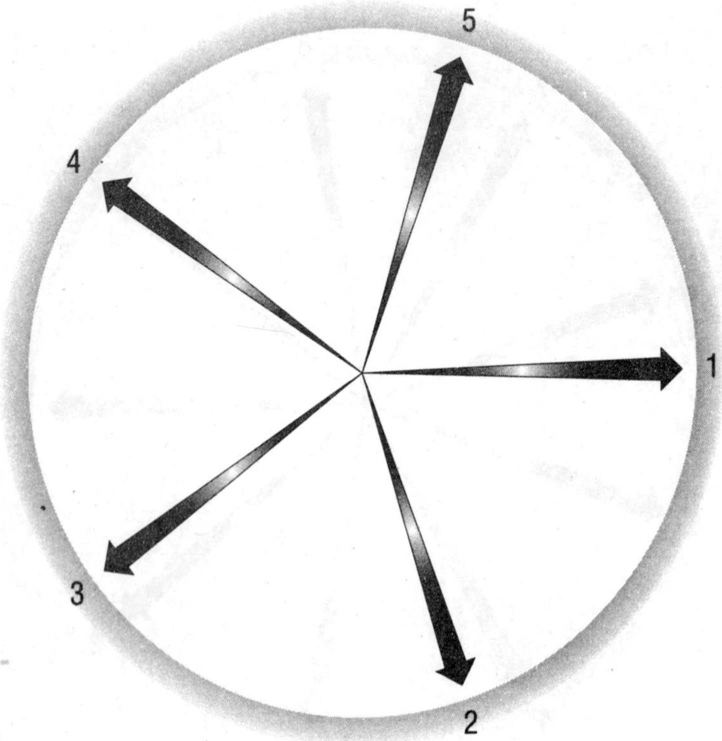

1. *Etheric body*
2. *Emotional body*
3. *Mental body*
4. *Spiritual body*
5. *Error*

Pendulum Table 4

Main Chakras

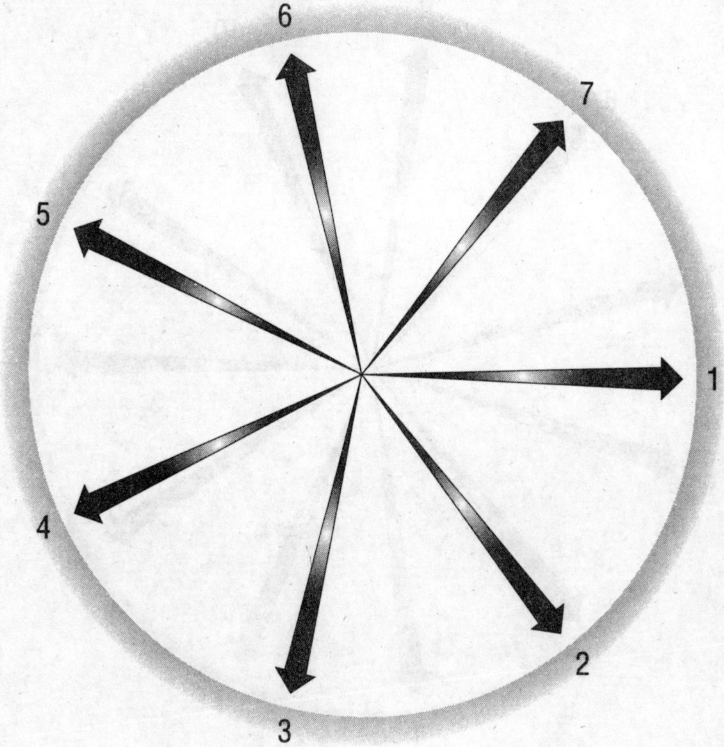

1. *Root chakra*
2. *Sexual chakra*
3. *Solar plexus chakra*
4. *Heart chakra*
5. *Throat chakra*
6. *Forehead chakra*
7. *Error*

Secondary Chakras

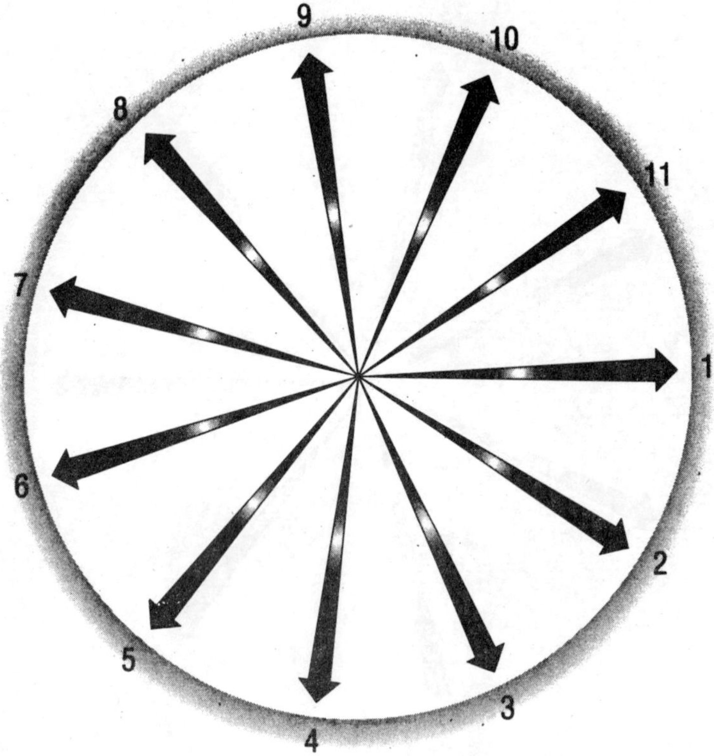

1. *Yin/yang*	6. *Sole*
2. *Nutrition/ responsiblity*	7. *Error*
3. *Elbow*	8. *Right*
4. *Palm*	9. *Both*
5. *Knee*	10. *Left*
	11. *Error*

Pendulum Table 6

The Bioenergetic Armor Rings

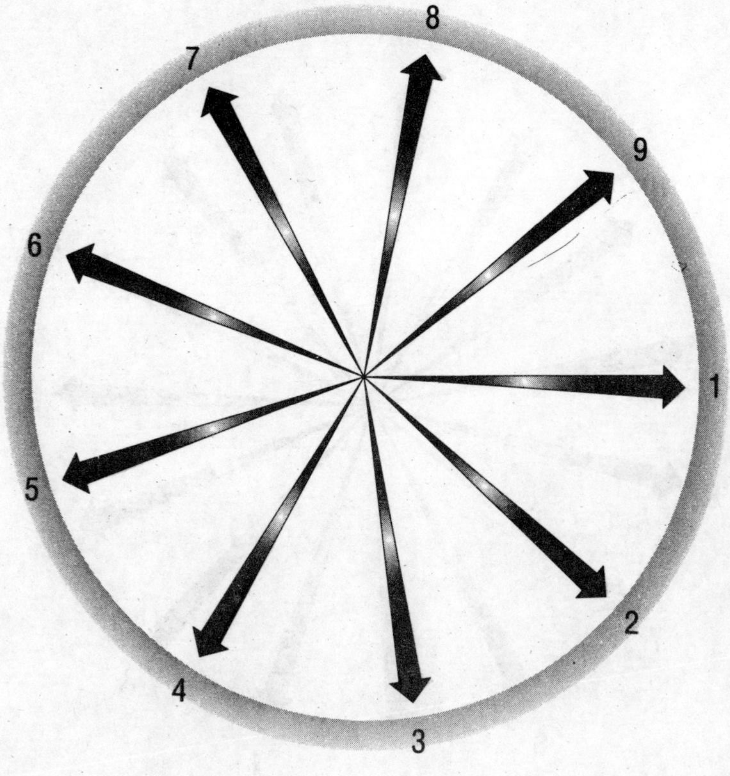

1. *1st Armor Ring*
2. *2nd Armor Ring*
3. *3rd Armor Ring*
4. *4th Armor Ring*
5. *5th Armor Ring*
6. *6th Armor Ring*
7. *7th Armor Ring*
8. *8th Armor Ring*
9. *Error*

Pendulum Table 7

Main Meridians

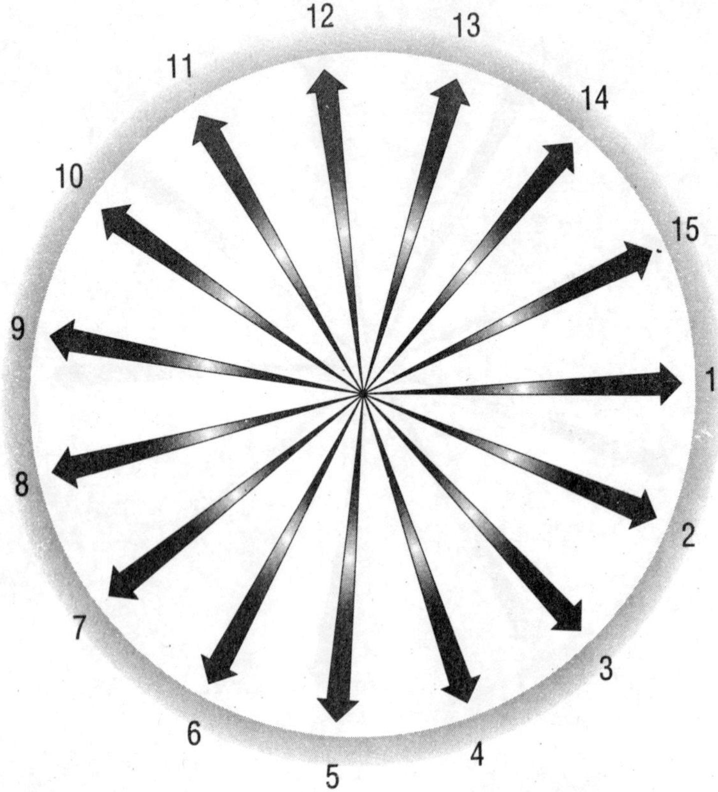

1. *Liver meridian*
2. *Heart meridian*
3. *Spleen-pancreas meridian*
4. *Lung meridian*
5. *Kidney meridian*
6. *Circulation-sex meridian*
7. *Gallbladder meridian*
8. *Small intestine meridian*
9. *Stomach meridian*
10. *Large intestine meridian*
11. *Bladder meridian*
12. *Triple warmer meridian*
13. *Conception vessel*
14. *Governor's vessel*
15. *Error*

Pendulum Table 8

Main Energy Organs

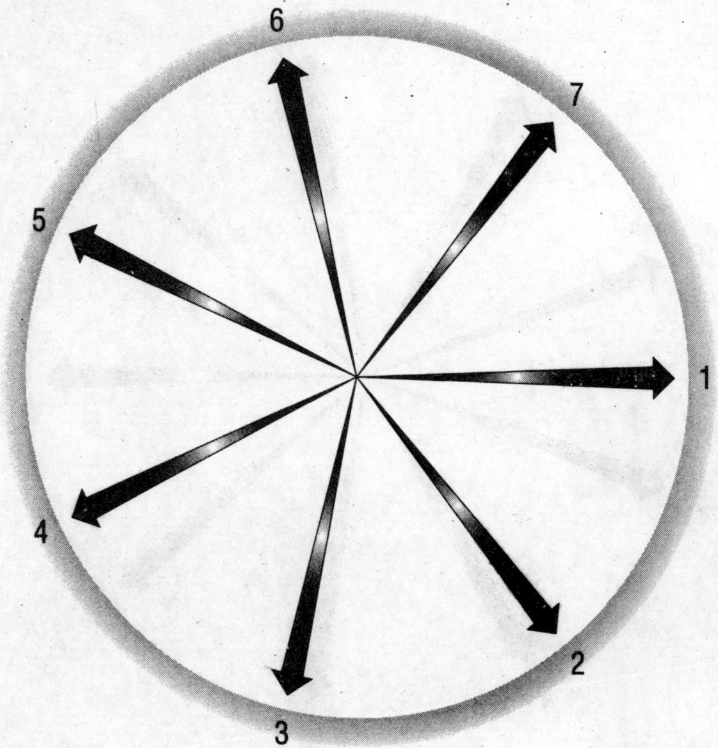

1. *Heart*
2. *Kidneys*
3. *Liver*
4. *Error*
5. *Lungs*
6. *Spleen*
7. *Error*

Pendulum Table 9

Colors

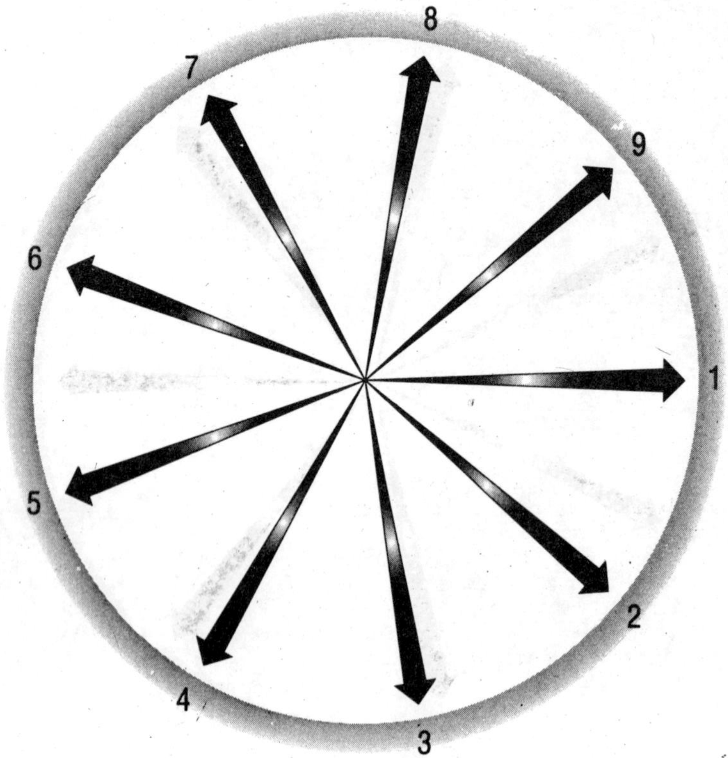

1. *Black*
2. *Red*
3. *Orange*
4. *Yellow*
5. *Green*
6. *Blue*
7. *Violet*
8. *White*
9. *Error*

Pendulum Table 10

Percentile Share of an Energy/Organ (in a disorder)

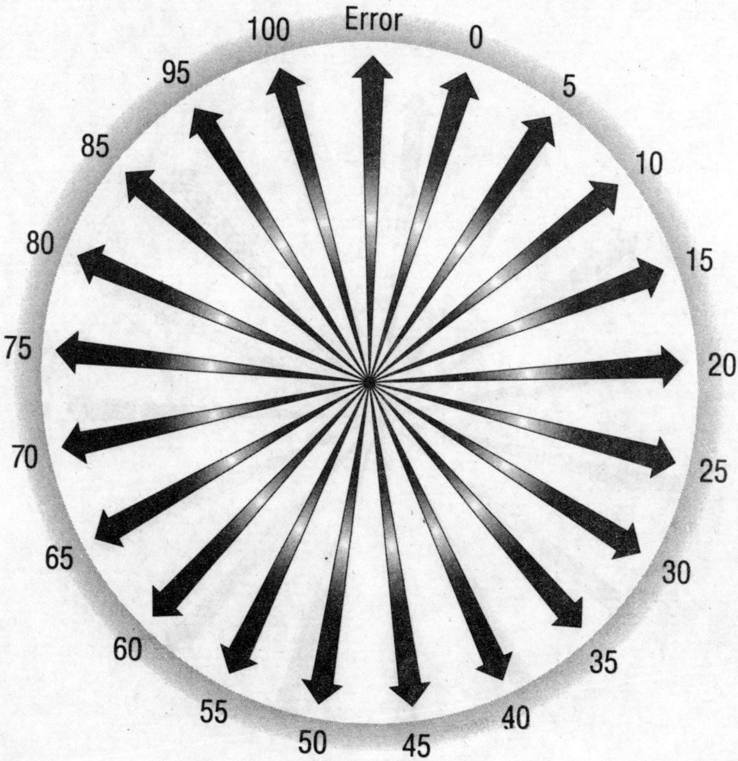

Pendulum Table 11

Some Frequent Causes of Blocks I

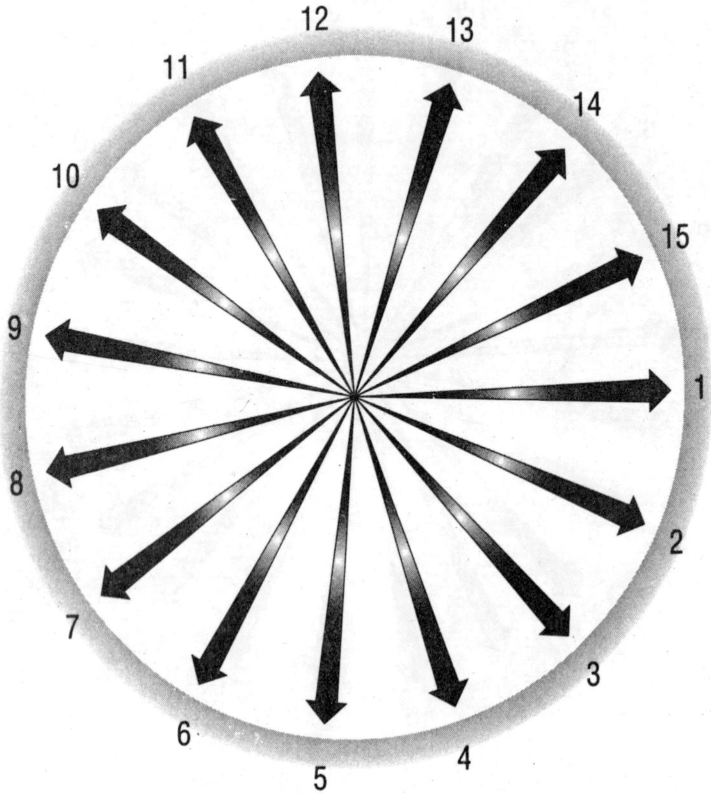

1. *Rejects personal responsibility*
2. *Inharmonious approach to sexuality*
3. *Inharmonious approach to aggression*
4. *Lives from own will*
5. *Not connected with heaven*
6. *Not grounded*
7. *Table II*
8. *Confuses power with love*
9. *Karmic*
10. *Helper syndrome*
11. *Wants to suffer*
12. *Can't accept anything*
13. *Lives outside life plan*
14. *For your own entry*
15. *Error*

Pendulum Table 12

Some Frequent Causes of Blocks II

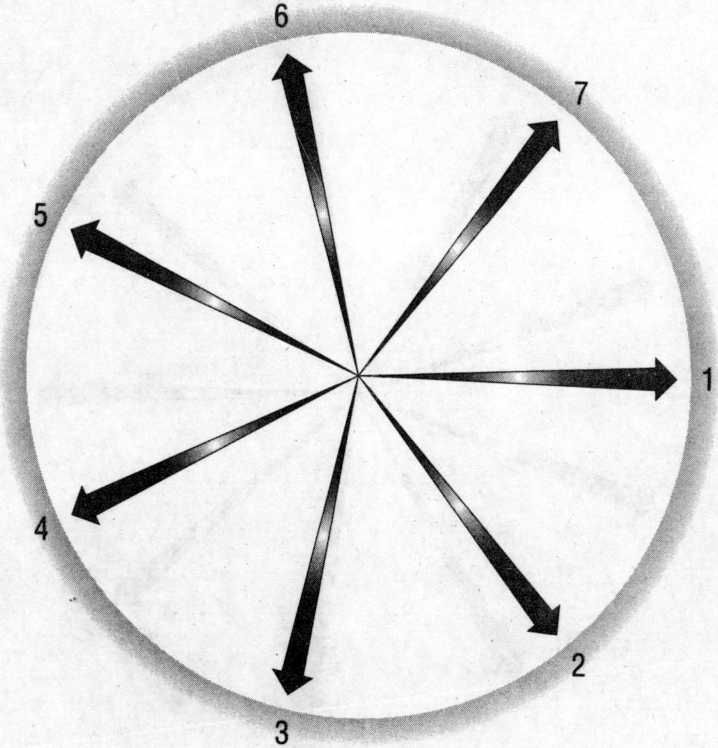

1. *Can't forgive/forget*
2. *Rejects part of self*
3. *Pays too little attention to feelings*
4. *Contemplates too little*
5. *Too theoretic*
6. *Too much black/white thinking*
7. *Error*

Pendulum Table 13

Support of Reading By

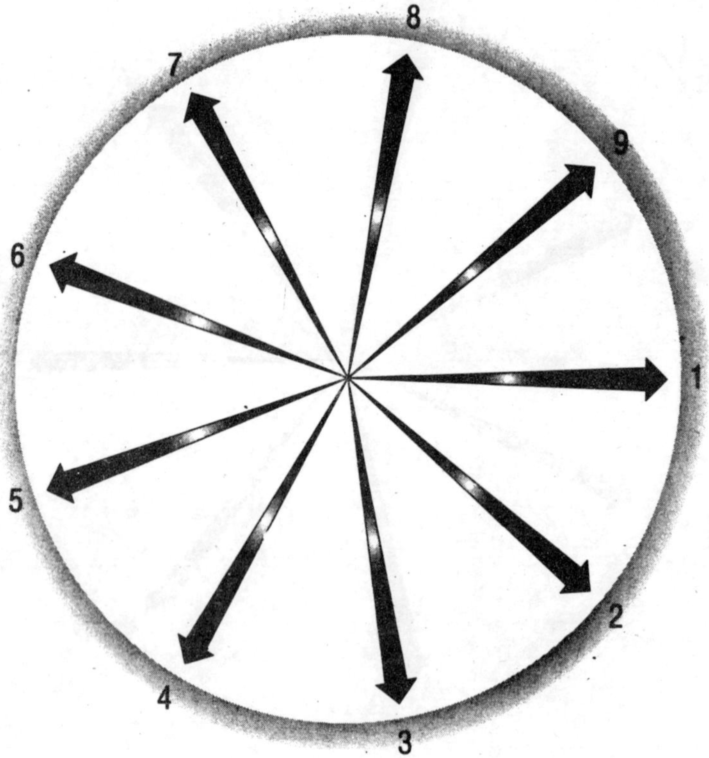

1. *Cards of Power*
2. *Conversation*
3. *Error*
4. *Using the pendulum*
5. *I Ching*
6. *OH Cards*
7. *Runes*
8. *Tarot*
9. *Error*

Pendulum Table 14

Simple Self-Help Measures

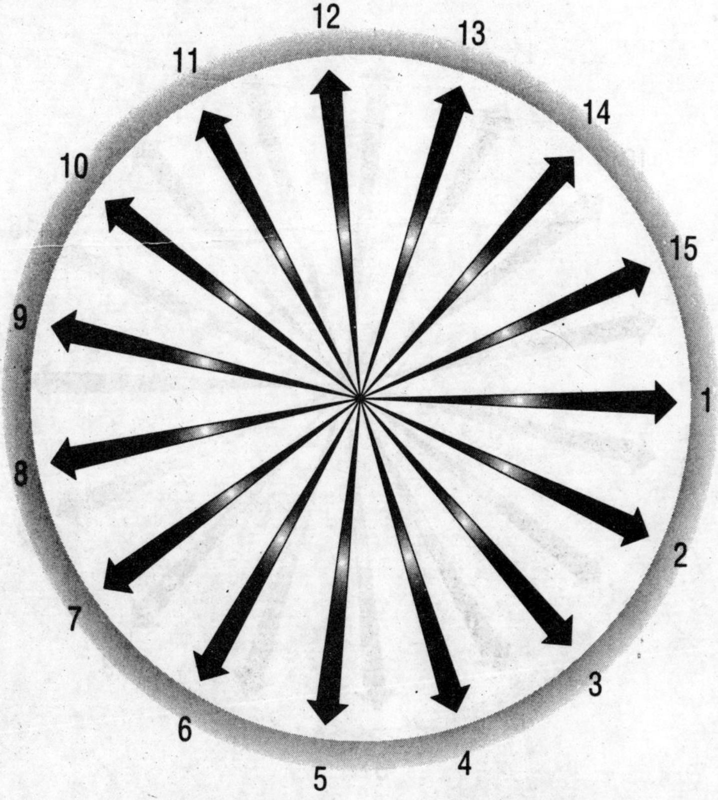

1. Bach Flowers
2. Drink more
3. Rest
4. Massage
5. Herbal therapy
6. Meditation
7. Aromatherapy
8. More exercise
9. Gemstone therapy
10. Color therapy
11. Reiki I
12. Different diet
13. Reiki II
14. Error
15. Error

Pendulum Table 15

For Your Own Entries

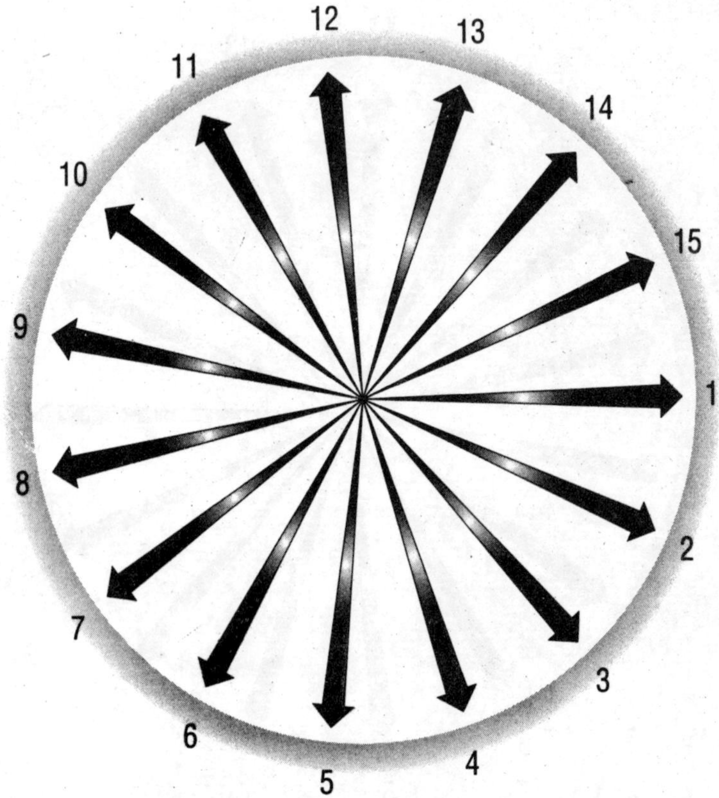

Energram Record

The following record can be photocopied. Please enlarge to standard paper size for your own use.

Date: ____________________

Name: ____________________

Topic: ____________________

1. Color generally in foreground:

____

2. Color generally in background:

____

1A: Aura ____________________

1B: Main chakras ____________________

1C: Secondary chakras ____________________

2A: Aura ____________________

2B: Main chakras ____________________

2C: Secondary chakras ____________________

Especially conspicuous:

____

Rune:
Topic: ____________________

Cards of Power:
Topic: ____________________

I Ching Hexagram:
Topic: ____________________

BLOCKS—organic—

Armor rings	Weakest	Strongest
Ring 1	☐	☐
Ring 2	☐	☐
Ring 3	☐	☐
Ring 4	☐	☐
Ring 5	☐	☐
Ring 6	☐	☐
Ring 7	☐	☐

BLOCKS—energetic—

Blocks	Weakest	Strongest
Aura	☐	☐
Main chakras	☐	☐
Secondary chakras	☐	☐
Meridians	☐	☐
Energy organs	☐	☐
Armor rings	☐	☐

New appointment:

____

Done on:

____

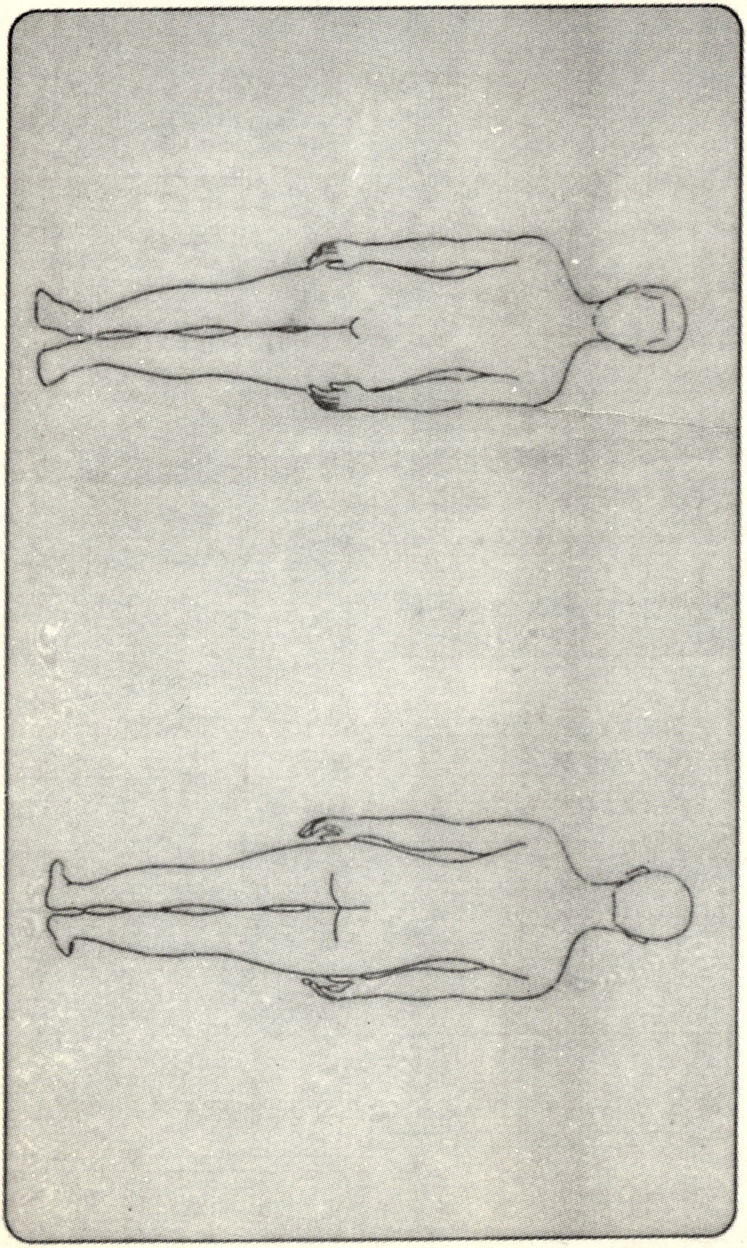

Appendix IV

Recommended Reading

The following literature recommendations are organized according to topic. I have tried to select from the diversity of publications those that are, in my opinion, best suited in terms of presenting comprehensive information about one area. This doesn't mean that I agree with everything written in the books listed. I think it's important to hear a number of different opinions in order to form one's own opinion as a result. In any case, that's how I learn best. Who can claim to know the truth alone?! However, in making this selection I've placed much value on naming trustworthy and reliable authors. I hope you enjoy looking through these books, comparing them, and learning from them!

AIKIDO

KI—A Practical Guide for Westerners by William Reed, Foreword by Koichi Tohei, Japan Publications, Inc. A good book about practical KI work and the life philosophy of the martial art of Aikido. Many exercises and thought-provoking ideas.

ALTERNATIVE HEALING METHODS

The "Gift" of Healing by Gerald Loe, Toe of the Mountain Publishing. A good, exciting book for becoming acquainted with serious spiritual healing, although I find it indispensable to learn from an experienced teacher. Knowledge from books is adequate for information purposes, but not for the practice!

Bach Flower Therapy by Mechthild Scheffer, Healing Arts Press.

Aromatherapy to Heal & Tend the Body by Robert Tisserand, Lotus Press. The fundamentals of aromatherapy with examples of applications and recipes. Good for beginners.

Enchanting Scents (Secrets of Aromatherapy) by Monika Jünemann, Lotus Light/Shangri-La. Psychological effects of scents, described in an interesting and detailed manner.

The Metamorphic Technique, Principles and Practice by Gaston Saint-Pierre & Debbie Boater, Element Books Ltd./UK.

The Complete Reiki Handbook by Walter Lübeck, Lotus Light/Shangri-La.

Reiki—Way of the Heart by Walter Lübeck, Lotus Light/Shangri-La.

Rainbow Reiki by Walter Lübeck, Lotus Light/Shangri-La. Rainbow Reiki is a new system based upon traditional Reiki but expanded with techniques for contacting spirits, channeling information from subtle dimensions, producing powerful Reiki Essences from, for example, plants, gemstones, and spiritual beings, activating crystals and using them with special Rainbow Reiki healing mandalas, advanced aura/chakra energy work, and much more.

Reiki For First Aid by Walter Lübeck, Lotus Light/Shangri-La. Reiki treatment as accompanying therapy for more than 40 types of health disorders. With a supplement of natural-healing methods and special Reiki healing diet.

Reiki Fire by Arjawa Frank Petter, Lotus Light/Shangri-La. New well-researched information about the origin of the Reiki power and Dr. Usui's true five principles for spiritual living. Very important to anyone who is interested in Reiki.

Reiki—Universal Life Energy by Shalila Sharamon/Bodo Baginski, Life Rhythm. This was the orignal book about Reiki. It reflects the atmosphere created by Reiki and is particularly recommended for beginners.

CHAKRAS

The Chakra Handbook by Shalila Sharamon/Bodo Baginski, Lotus Light/Shangri-La. An excellent book about the function of the seven main chakras with many exercises, classification tables, and thought-provoking ideas.

Hands of Light—A Guide to Healing Through the Human Energy Field by Barbara Ann Brennan, Bantam Books/NY

Inner Bridges by Fritz Frederick Smith, Humanic Publications. Much important information and correlations within the human energy system, rarely found in other sources.

The Body of Light by John Mann & Lar Short, Globe Press Books/NY. A comprehensive description of the human energy system in the various traditions (Buddhism, Hinduism, Taoism, and others). Very interesting and worth reading!

CHINESE MEDICINE

Traditional Acupuncture: The Law of the Five Elements by Duianne M. Connelly, The Center for Traditional Acupuncture/Maryland. A good portrayal of the Chinese five element system. Interesting and easy to understand.

Life Energy by John Diamond, M.D., Paragon House Not directly Chinese, but based on the meridian system. Interesting classifications and practical methods of checking how the meridians are charged.

Awaken Healing Energy Through Tao, Mantak Chia, Aurora Press/NY.

I CHING

The I Ching Workbook by R. L. Wing, Doubleday & Co. The ancient Chinese wisdom and oracle book is depicted by the author in a form that's modern, concise, and understandable for beginners.

The Taoist I Ching by Thomas Cleary, Shambala Publications/Boston. A profound translation for advanced students who would like to study this ancient book of wisdom more intensively.

KAHUNA MAGIC

Growing into Light by M. F. Long, DeVorss & Co. A classic work about the modern Kahuna method. An absorbing book containing much useful information.

Kahuna Healing by Serge King, Quest Books. Lots of information about Kahuna, written in a modern style with a very practice-oriented approach.

KINESIOLOGY

Brain-Gym by P. & G. Dennison, self-published. Holistic improvement of abilities to learn and concentrate through applied kinesiology.

One Brain: Workshop Book by Gordon S. Stokes, Three in One Concepts Inc./CA. An extensive introduction to the theory and practice of one of the most important schools of applied kinesiology.

MEDITATION

Zen Mind, Beginners Mind by Shunryu Suzuki, John, Weatherhill, Inc./ New York.

PERSONALITY DEVELOPMENT

Back to One by Sheldon B. Kopp, Science & Behavior Books Inc./CA. Fundamentals of modern psychotherapy in a synthesis with Eastern wisdom interpreted in a practical way.

Embracing Each Other, Hal & Sidra Stone, New World Library/CA. Being happy with each other as a couple without neglecting the relationship to oneself.

Everyone's a Coach by Ken Blanchard & Don Shula, Harper Business/NY. Success strategies of top athletes can also help "average people" achieve extraordinary performance and a positive attitude toward life.

PSYCHOSOMATIC MEDICINE/THERAPY

Body, Self & Soul-Sustaining Integration by J. L. Rosenberg, Humanics Publ. Group/GA. An outstanding book about spiritual, body-oriented therapy. Practical and informative.

Job's Body by Deane Juhan, Station Hill Press/NY. A standard work of body therapy. Extensive in detail yet still exciting to read.

RADIESTHESIA

The Pendulum Healing Handbook by Walter Lübeck, Lotus Light/Shangri-La. A practical guide to using the pendulum. Tips for selecting the right pendulum for you, measuring various types of disruptive rays, working with the pendulum tables, and many practical exercises for developing the ability to use the pendulum. With a very extensive collection of pendulum tables in the form of a pendulum oracle.

TAI CHI CHUAN

Advanced Tai Chi Form Instructions by Cheng Man-Ch'ing, Sweet Chi Press/NY.

There Are No Secrets—Professor Cheng Man-Ch'ing and His Tai Chi Chuan, Wolfe Lowenthal, North Atlantic Books/CA.

These are two standard works on Tai Chi Chuan. Deep philosophical insights are translated into practical ways of developing the personality in everyday life.

TANTRA

Sexual Secrets by Nik Douglas & Penny Slinger, Destiny Books/NY. An aesthetically presented work on the secrets of the spiritual art of love. Almost all important components of classic and modern Tantra are explained in a graphic way.

About the Author—Walter Lübeck

Walter Lübeck, born on February 17, 1960 (Aquarius, Asc. Sagittarius) lives in Weserbergland/Germany, a mystical landscape with many ancient power places that inspire him both personally and professionally. He has been interested in esotericism, parapsychology, and methods of alternative healing since his youth. His work is based on various forms of training, such as traditional Western paths of initiation, the Usui System of Reiki, Neurolinguistic Programming (NLP), Silva Mind Control, Tai Chi, and Asiatic forms of meditation. Walter Lübeck works in Germany, Austria, and Switzerland as a seminar head.

His work focuses on the following areas: Rainbow Reiki, which he has developed; energy and oracle work with the I Ching; reading auras and chakras; holistic training in money and success; Three-Rays Meditation; and spiritual NLP. The abundant results of his research are documented in fifteen books, which have been translated into ten languages, a teaching video on the topic of Rainbow Reiki, and diverse articles in specialized magazines.

Walter Lübeck orients himself toward three principles: support of individual responsibility; development of the ability to love, and consciousness expansion. His goal is the concrete betterment of the quality daily life through spiritual knowledge, thereby contributing toward bringing human beings, God, and nature into greater harmony. Not only have increasing numbers of Reiki Masters become associated with his Reiki-Do Institute and the work group Rainbow Reiki International, established several years ago—medical professionals and psychotherapists with a holistic approach to their work are also participating in the international healing and development network.

About the Author—Walter Lübeck

[illegible]